Parkinson's Disease
300 Tips for
Making Life Easier

Parkinson's Disease 300 Tips for Making Life Easier

Shelly Peterman Schwarz

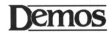

Demos Medical Publishing, Inc., 386 Park Avenue South,
New York, New York 10016

Library of Congress Cataloging-in-Publication Data

Schwarz, Shelley Peterman.
  Parkinson's disease : 300 tips for making life easier / Shelley Peterman Schwarz.
    p. ; cm.
Includes index.
  ISBN 1-888799-65-X (pbk.)
  1. Parkinson's disease—Popular works.
  [DNLM: 1. Parkinson Disease—rehabilitation—Popular Works.   2. Activities of Daily Living—Popular Works.   WL 359 S411z2002]   I. Title: Three hundred tips for making life with Parkinson's disease easier.   II. Title.
  RC382 S3825   2002
  362.1'96833—dc21

                                                                2002000363

Made in Canada

Dear Readers

Dear Readers,

This book is written for you because you or someone you care about has Parkinson's disease (PD). *300 Tips for Making Life with Parkinson's Disease Easier* is filled with tried and true tips, techniques, shortcuts, and resources that will help people coping with Parkinson's disease. These simple, inexpensive hints will save you time and energy, lessen your frustration, and promote safety and independence.

The information for this book was gathered from two sources: (1) interviews with more than 100 people living with Parkinson's disease, people who care for people with PD, and healthcare professionals; and (2) my own personal experiences living with multiple sclerosis (MS), which is, like Parkinson's disease, a chronic, degenerative, and incurable illness.

Did you find it a shock when you or your friend or loved one was diagnosed with PD? When I was diagnosed with MS more than 20 years ago, it changed my life forever. My diagnosis came after years of minor but ever-present complaints. Frankly, when the diagnosis came, I was relieved that there was a name for my seemingly unrelated symptoms. And, for a few years, I tried to ignore the disease and pass as "normal." Eventually, my limitations became more serious and I had to come to terms with the fact that I had a progressively degenerative disease that was impacting not just me but my family and friends as well.

Over the years I've learned to incorporate into my life some basic concepts that have helped me immensely, and I've learned thousands of simple time- and energy-saving tips that make a big difference in the quality of my life. Talking to others with chronic illnesses or disabilities has taught me a lot about survival and the human spirit and how strong and resilient people can be. We may not have a choice about having an illness, but we do have a choice in the way we react to it.

Receiving a diagnosis such as Parkinson's disease can be distressing, and adjusting to the effects of the disease can be difficult, but you can still lead a remarkably unlimited life if you put your mind to it. By adapting your routine, making your home more accessible, and keeping a positive outlook, you have the power to take control of your life and rise above the challenges of PD.

This book features tips to help you streamline daily activities, find ways to stay involved and in touch, and discover local, state, and national resources to make your life easier. The book is arranged in categories of daily activities for easy reference. At the beginning of each chapter, I share some of the insights and observations people with PD have made while living with this disease.

It is my hope that learning how other people deal with the challenges of Parkinson's disease will help you keep a positive attitude on your journey. I also hope the book will allow you to face the future with a sense of empowerment and control over the illness.

If, after reading this book, you would like to share your own Making Life Easier tips, or you just want to talk, I can be reached at

http://www.MakingLifeEasier.com

and

help@MakingLifeEasier.com.

I wish you the best on your journey.

Shelley Peterman Schwarz

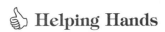 Helping Hands

Throughout this book you will notice tips with the **Helping Hands** designation. These tips are especially for people who provide care and support for people with PD.

Contents

CHAPTER 1

Basic Concepts for Living with Parkinson's Disease

Being diagnosed with a chronic progressive illness like Parkinson's disease (PD) changes your life forever. Don't give in or give up to the disease! Today is a very hopeful time for people with PD. I hope these thought and observations will help you.

STAYING POSITIVE WHILE LIVING WITH PARKINSON'S DISEASE

1. **Learn about your illness.** Don't be afraid to read about Parkinson's disease or talk to others who have it. Remember that no two cases are exactly alike and no one can predict exactly how the disease will progress or affect *you*. Likewise, no two people respond exactly the same to treatments and medications. Gathering information about your illness will also empower you to make informed decisions about your medical care and the treatment options open to you.

1

See if there is a Parkinson's disease or movement disorder clinic in your area. There have been many advances in the treatment of PD, and general neurologists may not be able to keep up to date on all areas of neurology. A specialist can confirm your diagnosis, review your medications, and consult with your primary care doctor on your treatment.

Once you understand your illness, you are in a better position to take responsibility for your healthcare.

2. **Look for ways to reduce your stress level and put yourself and your needs first.** This is not selfish or self-centered. You must take care of yourself first. You are the authority regarding your own body. Rest when you're tired. Be protective about how you spend your time and energy. Parkinson's disease uses a great deal of one's physical energy. Coping and adapting take a great deal of emotional and mental energy. Do the things that are important to you and your family. Give yourself permission to say "No," and don't feel guilty. When you are feeling better, you can say "Yes."

3. **It may be difficult, but try not to be self conscious about the visible symptoms of your Parkinson's disease.** Work around the problems. If you are self-conscious about the way you walk, consider using a wheelchair. If hand tremors make it difficult to eat with utensils and you are embarrassed to eat out in a restaurant, order foods you can eat with your hands and ask the waitress to put each item on a separate plate or bowl; that way your tremors are less likely to

knock food off the plate. Don't let your visible symptoms of PD diminish the enjoyment you get from spending time with your family and friends.

4. **Keep your sense of humor!** Having trouble walking, being unable to talk as loudly as you want, or giving up driving are not particularly funny. However, try to put a humorous spin on everyday observations and situations. For example, if you use a wheelchair, you might look at it this way: You always have a place to sit and a pair of shoes lasts you 20 years. Remember, laughter is a great stress reducer.

5. **Surround yourself with caring, loving, and nurturing family members, friends, neighbors, and co-workers.** Give yourself permission to eliminate people and activities that drain your energy. Be honest with your family and friends if you're having a bad day. Explain that you may feel terrible in the morning but fine in the afternoon. Don't expect people to know what you are feeling unless you tell them.

6. **Tell people about your illness.** At any age, it can be difficult to share your feelings with your friends. And it can be especially difficult if you're diagnosed with PD when you're young. Your friends may not know what PD is and may not know what to say or what to do. So tell them. Also tell your hair stylist, dentist, and salespeople (as appropriate) that you may shake, lose your balance, move slowly, or have difficulties speaking because of PD. Ask for their help when you need it. People feel good when they can do something for someone else.

You might also want to keep a few informational brochures in your purse or wallet because you never know who might be interested in learning more about Parkinson's disease.

7. **Try to keep a positive attitude** even though it can be extremely difficult as your symptoms change and the effectiveness of medications plays havoc with your life. It's perfectly natural to mourn the loss of function and independence for a brief time, but try not to get stuck and wallow in self-pity and isolate yourself from friends.

    If you experience a combination of these problems — loss of appetite, feelings of sadness, difficulty sleeping, loss of your sense of humor, a sense of hopelessness, or just feel down in the dumps — you may be suffering from clinical depression. Please! Tell your doctor. Even though you have every right to be depressed about your diagnosis, depression is a treatable condition. A combination of antidepressants and/or psychotherapy can help lift your spirits and give you renewed energy to keep that all-important positive attitude.

    Remember: Your family and friends are not trained professionals. In fact, they also may be hurting because of your diagnosis. Perhaps they, too, could benefit from talking to someone about their fears and frustrations.

    Listen to audiotapes and/or read books that promote positive thinking and deliver a healing message. The public library and bookstores offer an array of these materials.

8. **Set priorities and focus on tasks that must be done.** Tackle one job at a time. Break down activ-

ities into a series of smaller steps and ask others to assist you with the difficult portions of the task. Avoid working or sitting for long periods in the same position. Move around periodically.

9. **Allow extra time to do everything from eating, drinking, and dressing to walking, talking, and writing.** Recognize that everything seems to take longer when you have Parkinson's disease. You'll also find that simple tasks most people take for granted, like swallowing saliva, chewing food, changing facial expressions, and projecting your voice, now require conscious thought.

   Plan to do activities around the times your medication gives you the most benefit. Mornings are often a better time of day to exercise and work because you are not as fatigued as in the afternoon. Even though you may get fatigued during the day, be careful not to nap too much; otherwise, sleeping at night might be difficult. Taking a short nap after lunch can be revitalizing, but try to limit your daytime sleep so your nighttime sleep can be more restful.

10. **Consider attending a local PD support group,** no matter what your age. Support group members understand your struggles because they face or have faced the same challenges. To find a Parkinson's disease support group in your community, see the Resources section at the end of this chapter or consult the Yellow Pages of your telephone book.

   If you are reluctant to attend a PD support group because you will see others with advanced cases and you don't think you can handle that, talk on the phone with others who have PD. Or start a smaller group for lunch or coffee. Being with others who have PD may alleviate fears rather than worsen them. It is encouraging to see people with PD still driving, working, and caring for their families.

11. **Understand that it is common to have fluctuations in your mobility and energy levels during the day.** Often these fluctuations coincide with when you take your medications, with the most fatigue and the least mobility coming as the medication wears off.

12. **Be willing to change the way you do things.** Remain flexible. Compromise. Accept the help that is offered and accept that there is more than one way to wash the dishes, put on clothes, or get from here to there. Practice patience — with yourself and others.

13. **Ask your doctor to prescribe evaluations by an occupational therapist (OT) and physical therapist (PT).** An OT will help you discover new ways of doing simple, everyday tasks like dressing, eating, and cooking. He or she can show you how to simplify your work and daily activities and conserve your energy. A PT will help you with mobility and home accessibility. Ask for a home evaluation and ask the OT and PT to make suggestions for making your home and daily activities safer, more accessible, and easier to manage.

14. **Always try out any mobility equipment before you buy it.** That includes canes, walkers,

manual and electric wheelchairs, transport chairs (all four of the wheels are the same size), and three-wheeled scooter wheelchairs. Check out the size, weight, and ease of operation. If someone will be pushing your wheelchair, explain to that person about "courtesies of the road," including speed, cornering, handling leg rests, backing into elevators, and going up and down curbs, etc.

If you are considering purchasing a 3- or 4-wheeled scooter or wheelchair, find one that is easy to transport. Some chairs are lightweight and disassemble easily. Others come with trunk lifts that pick up the chair and put it into the car with minimal physical effort. Certain car companies offer ramps where the wheelchair user simply drives up the ramp and stays in the chair without transferring

15. **Make exercise part of your life** and it will improve your quality of life. Exercise does not reverse or delay the symptoms of PD, but it *does* help you make full use of your potential. It also helps prevent complications, such as contractures of rigid, poorly moving limbs. Walking, range-of-motion exercises, and simple stretching regimens can do wonders for your energy level, strength, and general feelings of well-being. Tai chi can help with balance, as well as providing a time for quiet meditation. Your doctor or physical therapist can suggest an exercise program that will help keep you active. Ask several friends and/or family members to be your workout buddies so you can have daily encouragement to adhere to your program.

BASIC CONCEPTS FOR PEOPLE WHO HELP PEOPLE WITH PD

👍 **Helping Hands**

16. Periodically, the person with PD may experience hallucinations or delusions. It may be helpful to say, "I'm sure you really see the (little girl) but it's really the medication (or the Parkinson's disease) that's causing you to see (her). I'll call the doctor and see how we can make (her) disappear." Then redirect the person and say something like, "Let's get a glass of ice tea. Come and help me." Or explain that you're talking about what to get Mary for her birthday and ask, "What do you think she'd like?"

👍 **Helping Hands**

17. **Be encouraging.** Whether it's getting the person with Parkinson's disease to exercise, eat, dress, or do any other activity, have a positive, patient, and encouraging attitude. Allow the person with PD to do as much for himself or herself as possible. Squelch the tendency to jump up and do a task because you can do it faster and more easily than the person with PD. Also, encourage him or her to eat as much as possible independently before offering your assistance.

👍 **Helping Hands**

18. **Expect the person with Parkinson's disease to participate in daily activities as much as he or she can,** such as setting the table, folding laundry, and putting groceries away.

☝ Helping Hands

19. **Give verbal cues when necessary:** "Walk with me to the bedroom." Talk the person with Parkinson's disease through activities, like dressing and bathing. "Let's put on your shirt. Help me button your shirt. Let's tuck in your shirt and button your pants." Be patient and encouraging to minimize the stress of the situation.

☝ Helping Hands

20. **Encourage the person with Parkinson's disease to attend a support group meeting.** If that's not possible, try to arrange a one-on-one get together with another person with PD. If speech problems are not a factor, these "meetings" can be over the phone. For yourself, you might want to consider finding a caregivers' support group.

☝ Helping Hands

21. **Contact the local fire department about any special needs the person with Parkinson's disease might have should a fire emergency occur.** The information will be noted and in an emergency, the dispatcher will be able to tell the firefighters where to look for the person needing assistance, (i.e., which apartment, which bedroom), and what special equipment or rescue procedures might be necessary. Communities will vary as to how they record and retrieve this information so even if your community has the 911 emergency service, it is still important to contact your *local* fire department before tragedy strikes. (In some communities information

between the fire, police, and emergency medical services is not shared, so readers should contact each agency independently.)

RESOURCES

22. **Organizations and Web sites to help you and your family learn about PD:**

American Parkinson's Disease Association, Inc.
1250 Hylan Blvd., Ste. 4B
Staten Island, NY 10305-1946
(800) 223-2732
(718) 981-8001
(718) 981-4399 Fax
http://www.apdaparkinson.com

The National Parkinson Foundation, Inc.
Bob Hope Parkinson Research Center
1501 NW 9th Ave.Bob Hope Rd.
Miami, Florida 33136-1494
(305) 547-6666
(800) 327-4545(305) 243-4403 Fax
http://www.parkinson.org
mailbox@parkinson.org

Parkinson's Disease Foundation, Inc.
Parkinson's Disease Foundation
710 West 168th St.
New York, NY 10032-9982
(800) 457-6676
(212) 923-4700
(212) 923-4778 Fax
http://www.pdf.org
info@pdf.org

Parkinson's Action Network
300 N. Lee St., Ste. 500
Alexandria, VA 22314
(800) 850-4726
(703) 518-8877
(703) 518-0673 Fax
http://www.Parkinsonaction.org
info@parkinsonsaction.org

The Michael J. Fox Foundation for Parkinson's Research
Grand Central Station
P.O. Box 4777
New York, NY 10163
(800) 708-7644
http://www.michaeljfox.org

23. **Companies with Web sites that sell mobility equipment:**

Enrichments for Better Living
Sammons Preston
(An AbilityOne Corporation)
4 Sammons Ct.
Bolingbrook, IL 60440
(800) 323-5547
(800) 547-4333 Fax
http://www.sammonspreston.com
sp@sammonspreston.com

Access to Recreation, Inc.
8 Sandra Ct.
Newbury Park, CA 91320
(800) 634-4351
(805) 498-8186 Fax
http://www.accesstr.com

dkrebs@gte.net

Spinlife.com
1108 City Park Ave., Ste. 201
Columbus, OH 43206
(800) 850-0335
(614) 449-8123
(888) 873-6543 Fax
http://www.spinlife.com

Deming Designs Inc.
1090 Cobblestone Dr.
Pensacola, FL 32514
(850) 478 5765
(850) 476-3361 Fax
http://www.beachwheelchair.com
kmdeming@aol.com

Finders Medical Depot
Leaders in New and Used Medical Equipment
3401 N.W. 7th Street
Miami, FL 33125
(305) 644-1129
http://www.findersmedical.com

If you don't have Internet access at home, visit your local library and ask a librarian how to visit these sites.

CHAPTER 2

Making Your Home Safe and Accessible

You can make many simple and inexpensive modifications to your home to make it more accessible without spending lots of money to remodel or make extensive changes.

24. Some of the easiest changes you can make include the following:

   ◊ **Arrange furniture so that there are clear walking paths throughout the house.** Remove barriers such as magazine racks or footstools.

   ◊ **Place furniture in strategic locations** if you need to touch or hold onto it as you walk. Remove casters or wheels from furniture – objects that roll are unstable means of support.

   ◊ **Remove throw rugs,** which cause many trips and falls.

◊ **Increase lighting** by using the highest wattage light bulbs recommended. Purchase a gooseneck floor lamp from an office supply or furniture store. You can adjust the lamp and shine the light in any direction.

◊ **Replace glass shower doors with a lightweight shower curtain** for safety and convenience.

◊ **Store daily-use products like towels, dishes, food, spices, medications, and cleaning supplies between waist and eye level** to avoid reaching and bending, which can throw you off balance and lead to falls.

👍 Helping Hands

25. **Some people with PD propel themselves forward when they walk, such that they have difficulty stopping quickly enough to avoid walking into furniture or through a glass door.** If this is a problem for the person you help, strategically arrange the furniture so you create soft landings, like the arm of an upholstered couch. However, always consult the person with PD before rearranging any furniture so that he or she does not lose familiarity with the surroundings.

LIGHTING AND LIGHT SWITCHES

26. **Replace traditional light switches with rocker-panel switches** that require less fine motor control. They can be turned on or off by pressing with an arm, elbow, or palm of the hand. Rocker panel switches are available with built-in illumi-

nation, so you don't have to grope in a dark room to locate the switch. These are available at hardware and home-building supply stores.

27. **Purchase touch-sensitive lamps** if manipulating the small turn-screw on most lamps is difficult. To turn on a touch-sensitive lamp, you simply touch any metal on the base and the light goes on. Touch it a second time and the light goes off, or if you use a three-way bulb, the light gets brighter with each successive touch. Or purchase a converter kit that easily transforms a traditional lamp into a touch-sensitive one. The converter fits into the part where the bulb normally goes, and after you install a bulb, the lamp lights up when you touch it.

28. **Install motion detector light switches** in the basement, garage, and utility room. Motion detector switches are especially useful in areas where you often find your arms full (with laundry, groceries, etc.). The light turns on when you enter the room and turns off a few minutes after you leave. Or use photosensitive night-lights that automatically turn on at dusk.

SAFETY AND EMERGENCY PROVISIONS

29. **Put glow-in-the-dark tape or stickers on the handles of flashlights** so you can find them easily if your electricity goes out.

30. **If you have diminished sensitivity to temperature,** set your water heater's thermostat some-

where below 120 degrees Fahrenheit to avoid accidental scalding while bathing or washing.

31. **Install smoke and carbon monoxide detectors** upstairs and downstairs in your home. Having smoke detectors is important because of the loss of the sense of smell associated with Parkinson's disease. Having detectors for carbon monoxide, an odorless gas, is important in every home. Replace the batteries in these detectors once every year. Replace the detectors themselves every 5–10 years.

DOORS, DOORWAYS, AND DOORKNOBS

32. **Replace regular doorknobs with lever handles** or purchase a rubber lever that fits over any standard doorknob. Lever handles are easier to operate: just push down with your hand, arm, or elbow. Purchase lever handles at hardware or home building supply stores. Or wrap several rubber bands around the largest part of the doorknob to increase its diameter. It will be easier to grasp.

33. **You will need a minimum of 32 inches of clearance to get the average wheelchair through a doorway.** If you want to make your home doorways more wheelchair accessible, cut out the doorjamb molding starting from the floor and going up 3 to 4 feet. Removing this portion of the doorjamb will add an extra $1^1/2$ inches clearance for the wheelchair to get through. Or install offset hinges, which increase the door opening 2 to 3 inches, allowing the door to swing out and away

from the doorway opening. To find out how to purchase offset hinges, contact the resources listed in tip 73. Or, speak to a hospital occupational therapist or physical therapist about where to find these special hinges. The hinges cost about $10.

UNDER LOCK AND KEY

34. **Buy adaptive key devices that fit on regular keys and give better leverage turning keys.** Hardware, home health care, and medical supply stores and catalogs have different styles to choose from. Be sure to try them first to see which works the best for you.

35. **Keep duplicate full sets of keys in several places around the house** in case you misplace a set. Always try to put the keys you regularly use in one designated place (say, in a dish by the door most frequently used) to reduce the amount of time you spend hunting for them.

RAMPS, RAILINGS, STAIRS, AND GRAB BARS

👍 Helping Hands

36. **If the person with PD uses a wheelchair, install a ramp with a railing.** Be sure there is a level area in front of the door. A platform 5 feet wide and 3 feet long is recommended at the top of the ramp because it will be easier to unlock and open the door. Railing height above ramps is a matter of

personal preference. The average-sized person usually finds a height of 35–36 inches works well. If the person using the wheelchair is short, consider one that is 32-34 inches high. Railings should be installed on either side of the ramp. They should be $1^{1}/_{4}$ inches to $1^{1}/_{2}$ inches in diameter with $1^{1}/_{2}$ inches clearance from any obstruction such as a wall.

37. **Install hand railings on both sides of a stairway** wherever you have stairs, both inside and outside the house. Even if there are only one or two steps on the front porch, install handrails on both sides. It gives the dominant grip a firm hold going both up and down stairs, and you'll be more secure walking up and down those steps in inclement weather.

38. **Consider installing a railing along a long hallway in your home.**

39. **Place U-shaped handles at strategic doorway locations** to help you navigate through the doorway more easily. If you tend to fall backward when opening a door, drawer, or cabinet, you may want to install U-shaped handles at strategic locations by doors, drawers, or cabinets to help you keep your balance.

40. **Install grab bars wherever you need to hold onto something sturdy when transferring** from one place to another, such as to the toilet or tub. Decide where they will provide you with the most help. Leave a space the width of a clenched fist between the grab bar and the wall. Vinyl covered grab rails are better for grip and will absorb less heat.

When installing railings, U-shaped handles, or grab bars that will be used to support your weight, they must be securely anchored to wall studs. Get professional advice on the proper placement or hire a professional if you can't do the installation yourself.

41. **Install a floor-to-ceiling pole by the bed, toilet, living room chair, and dining room table.** These lightweight poles are held in place by controlled tension and require no special tools or structural changes for installation. You can use them as a steadying or balancing aid, and to help you get to a standing position.

THE KITCHEN

42. **If you plan to purchase new appliances,** consider buying a stove with a smooth top. It is much easier to clean. Buy a side-by-side refrigerator/freezer so you can store both frozen and refrigerated items at eye level.

43. **Store dishes, utensils, and food in locations closest to where you use them.** For instance, store dishes and glasses over the dishwasher or sink and hang pots and pans from hooks near the stove. Store frequently used items on the countertop or other convenient location. Avoid stacking or piling objects on top of each other. Label the drawers, cupboards, and cabinets in the kitchen with a description or a photo of the contents. This will cut down on the amount of time spent searching for items, especially if others frequently help you in the kitchen.

Place commonly used items on a turntable or lazy Susan in the center of the kitchen table or on a countertop. Also use a lazy Susan in a deep cabinet or cupboard so you can access the contents more easily.

44. **Look for a cutting board with a raised side,** or have wooden sides attached to your existing cutting board, to minimize spillage of diced food.

45. **Purchase a dustpan attached to a long handle** so you won't have to bend to use a dustpan. You can collect your floor sweepings while in a standing position.

THE BATHROOM

👍 Helping Hands

46. **Crisscross two pieces of adhesive tape over the bolt on the bathroom door.** Adults who are confused or have trouble operating a doorknob will not be able to lock themselves in the bathroom.

47. **If the bathroom doorway is too narrow to manage, remove the door.** Replace it with a tension rod and an opaque or black shower curtain liner. More clearance is helpful not just for wheelchair users, but also for those who use a walker or require assistance.

48. **Purchase a telescoping mirror** that either clamps to the side wall of the vanity or sits on

top of the vanity counter. Telescoping mirrors feature adjustable, swivel-type necks that can be moved to various positions easily. One side has a regular mirror and the other has a magnifying mirror, making it perfect for makeup application and shaving. Or consider installing mirror tiles at various heights on the bathroom walls.

49. **If you have separate controls for hot and cold water, consider installing wrist blades.** Wrist blades are wide, wing-type handles that can be operated by pushing with the forearm, wrist, or heel of the hand. These are available at most plumbing supply and hardware stores.

50. **Consider buying a removable showerhead on a flexible, hand-held extension hose.** They are fairly inexpensive and easy to install and make showering much easier, especially if you're sitting on a tub bench or shower chair. However, a hand-held shower nozzle can be very slippery and hard to grip when your hands are soapy. You'll have better control if you wind several rubber bands around the handle portion of the nozzle.

51. **Purchase an inexpensive resin or webbed outdoor chair or bench so you can sit while bathing or showering.** This will reduce your risk of slipping in the shower. Purchase these chairs at home supply or discount stores.

52. **A bath lift or bathtub transfer bench can make getting in and out of the tub much easier.** Bath lifts connect to a faucet or shower pipe and use

water pressure to lower you into and raise you out of the water. Bath lifts have hand controls so you can operate them without assistance. Some models are portable and lightweight so you can take them with you when you travel. Ask an occupational therapist about how to set up and adjust an appropriate bathtub transfer bench. For more information on bath lifts, see the Resources section at the end of this chapter.

53. **Purchase an adjustable portable toilet seat** to increase the height 3–7 inches and make it easier to get on and off the toilet. They are easy to attach to any toilet. Some raised seats provide armrests for added support. The models that come with a lock are the safest, because the lock prevents the seat from slipping off the toilet during a transfer. Buy a tote bag so you can take the seat with you and safely use bathrooms away from home.

THE BEDROOM

Setting Up the Bedroom

54. **The bed should be low enough for you to get in easily.** A good guideline is for the bed to be 22 inches high, but take your height into account. In general, if the bed is lower than knee height (like a futon), getting in and out will be difficult. If your bed is too low, set its legs on recessed wooden risers (blocks with holes cut into them to accommodate the bed legs). If your bed is too high, consult a carpenter to get the legs of the bed shortened.

55. **If nighttime incontinence creates occasional problems,** buy a plastic mattress cover at a discount store or a waterproof pad at a store where cribs or baby products are sold. The waterproof pad is a flat piece of flannel-like material that sits on the mattress in the middle of the bed and the fitted sheet goes on top of it. Or make the bed with two fitted sheets, placing a waterproof pad between the sheets. If the top sheet gets wet, remove it and the pad and you have a clean bed in a flash.

    If nighttime incontinence problems are chronic, consider wearing adult diapers.

    Be sure to discuss any incontinence problems with your doctor or a specialist.

Helping Hands

56. **If the person with PD spends lots of time in bed, make the bedroom a pleasant place to be for the both of you.** Orient the bed so that it faces a window. Bring in fresh flowers. Hang a frame or bulletin board with pictures of family and friends where it can be easily seen.

57. **Keep a water container with lid and drinking straw by the bedside.** Many sports bottles or children's cups come with a built-in fold-down straw. These drink containers are also good for travel because they won't spill if tipped over.

58. **Hang shoes by their laces or straps over the handle of your closet door** so you won't trip over them. In addition, you won't have to bend over to pick the shoes up.

Bed Rails and Bed Pulls

59. **Consider repositioning your bed against the wall** to make it more accessible. Install a grab bar on the wall alongside the bed, about ten inches higher than the mattress. Be sure to anchor the railing to studs in the wall so it will be secure. Or look into obtaining half bed rails that can be installed under the mattress. Installing such rails might eliminate the need for an expensive hospital bed with bed railings.

60. **Attach a bed pull to the grab bar or to the frame at the foot of your bed** to assist in turning over and getting out of bed. Use a nylon rope, or braid three pieces of tightly woven fabric together in a length that will reach from the base of the bed to your hand when lying down. It should be long enough for you to reach but still at arm's length for good leverage when you want to pull yourself out of bed. Tie a large wooden ring to the end to serve as a handhold. Then sew a binder clip (butterfly clip) near the ring so that the bed pull can be clamped to the bedding and remain within your reach. You can also attach a bed pull to the side of the bed to assist you in turning.

Turning Over in Bed

61. **Use satin bed sheets.** Their slippery surface makes it easier to turn over in bed. Flannel sheets make it more difficult to turn over than standard cotton percale sheets.

62. **Consider installing a trapeze or harness that hangs over the bed** so you can grab hold of it and lift and turn yourself.

63. **Place a long, sturdy cardboard box under the covers at the foot of the bed.** Elevating the covers will keep pressure off your feet and legs, and allow you to turn without getting tangled up in the bedding.

☝ **Helping Hands**

64. **If you need to move or reposition someone with Parkinson's disease in bed,** here is a technique you can use:

    ◊ Create a draw sheet by placing a flat sheet folded to fit from the person's chest to the thighs on the bed over the fitted sheet. This is what you'll use for leverage underneath the person.

    ◊ Grab the sheet with your palms up, count to three, and move/pull the person and draw sheet toward you.

    ◊ To do a two-person lift to reposition the person up or down in the bed, count to three and shift your body weight from the back to the front leg, keeping your arms and back in a locked position and together slide the person.

☝ **Helping Hands**

65. **Use baby monitors to hear a person with PD who is in bed.** The monitor's transmitter sits on the bedside table and the receiver goes in another room for remote listening. Some monitors have portable receivers so you can listen to the person as you move around the house.

👍 **Helping Hands**

66. **Help the person with PD feel relaxed in the bedroom** by implementing a few of these tips:

   ◊ **Give the person a back or leg massage.**

   ◊ **Keep a favorite blanket or pillow on the bed** for comfort and security. Don't purchase new linens without checking to see if the person with PD likes them. Bringing unfamiliar items into the environment can be very upsetting to people with PD who are confused or have dementia.

   ◊ **Use a night light or leave the bathroom or hall light on** to help keep the person with PD oriented to where he or she is.

FURNITURE AND FLOOR COVERINGS

67. **Walking or wheeling on carpet is easier if the carpet pile is very short.** It is easier still on wood, linoleum, or ceramic floors. However, bare floors and ceramic tiles can be slippery when wet, so use caution. You may want to consider changing the floor covering or surface.

68. **Use furniture that is sturdy and stable.** Generally the best sitting chair has a relatively straight back, a firm, shallow seat and armrests. Avoid low, heavily upholstered couches and chairs, as it is often difficult to rise from them without help. Sofas or chairs should be approxi-

mately 17 inches off the ground. The seat should be no lower than knee height. Add a firm cushion or attach risers to the chair legs to increase the height of the chair. For some, a comfortable, heavy rocking chair with armrests may help, as it can give you an extra boost when rising.

69. **To get out of a chair,** scoot forward to the edge of the seat, spread your feet apart, and rock back and forth to build up momentum.

RESOURCES

70. **The Guardian Safety Pole is a floor-to-ceiling pole that safely assists standing, sitting, climbing stairs, or transferring.** No tools are required for installation. Screw mechanism with padded bracket fits securely without marring surface. Its white, powder-coated, heavy gauge steel construction is attractive and durable.

   Sunrise Medical. North American Operations
   7477 E. Dry Creek Pkwy.
   Longmont, CO 80503
   (888) 333-2572
   (303) 218-4500
   (303) 218-4590 Fax
   http://www.sunrisemedical.com

71. **The Super Pole System is another modular support system that provides assistance with standing, transferring, or moving in bed.** The floor-to-ceiling pole is installed by simple jackscrew expansion.

Health Craft Products, Inc.
1230 Old Innes Rd., Unit 411
Ottawa, ON, Canada K1B 3V3
(888) 619-9992
(613) 744-3001
(613) 744-3008 Fax
http://www.healthcraftproducts.com

72. **Bathtub transfer benches and shower chairs come in a variety of sizes and styles.**

Sunrise Medical. North American Operations
7477 E. Dry Creek Pkwy.
Longmont, CO 80503
(888) 333-2572
(303) 218-4500
(303) 218-4590 Fax
http://www.sunrisemedical.com

73. **To locate items to help you with activities of daily living all around the house contact:**

Bed Handles™
4825 S. Tierney Drive
Independence, MO 64055
(800) 725-6903
(816) 478-4324 Fax
mailer@BedHandles.com
http://www.mailer@bedhandles.com

Access With Ease
P.O. Box 1150
Chino Valley, AZ 86323
(800) 531-9479
(520) 636-0292 Fax

http://www.shop.store.yahoo.com/capability/
index.html
kmjc@northlink.com

Easy Street
8 Springbrook Rd.
P.O. Box 146
Foxboro, MA 02035
(800) 959-EASY
http://www.easystreetco.com
support@easystreetco.com

Enrichments for Better Living
Sammons-Preston, Inc.
(A Subsidiary of Bissell Health Care Corp.)
P.O. Box 5071
Bollingbrook, IL 60440
(800) 323-5547
(800) 547-4333 Fax
http://www.sammonspreston.com
sp@sammonspreston.com

74. **For information on bath lifts,** contact Whitaker Stairway and Residence Elevators & Accessibility Lifts.

Whitaker
1 Odell Plaza, PO Box 1061
Yonkers, NY 10703
(800) 445-4387
(914) 423-4243
http://www.stairlift.com
info@stairlift.com

CHAPTER 3

Looking Good,
Feeling Better

When you look good, you tend to feel better. In this chapter, you'll find ways to streamline dressing so you'll have more time and energy to pursue other daily activities. But first, here are some basic concepts to keep in mind:

◊ **Dressing will be easier when your medications are working,** so plan to dress during your "on" time.

◊ **Allow enough time so that you don't feel rushed.** Gathering all your clothing items together before you start to dress will save steps and time. You may even find it helpful to lay your clothes out the night before. Then if you plan to wear something that needs to be hooked at the back, for example, you can ask for help before family members go off for the day.

◊ **If your balance is unsteady, sit on the bed or in a sturdy chair with armrests when you dress.** You may also want to sit when you do your hair, shave, or apply makeup.

GROOMING

75. **Substitute a wash mitt or soft sponge for the usual washcloth.** A wash mitt slips on the hand and can be easier to use than a washcloth. A sponge is lighter and easier to wring out. Lightweight cotton dishcloths are also easier to wring than terrycloth washcloths. A long-handled sponge or bath brush can be used to reach your legs, feet, and back without bending.

76. **Use soap-on-a-rope** to prevent the slips and falls that can occur in the shower when you bend to retrieve a dropped bar of soap. Hang the soap around your neck. If you can't find soap-on-a-rope at the drug store, make your own. Cut the leg from an old (clean) pair of pantyhose; place a bar of soap in the foot area; securely tie the top thigh area of the hose to the pipe behind the showerhead; then stretch the hose and use as a soap-on-a-rope (of hose). Or use shower gel on a bath pouf or sponge instead of a bar soap.

77. **Pour shampoo onto a sponge;** then rub the sponge on your hair. The shampoo is less likely to run into your eyes and there's no chance of dropping a slippery bottle in the tub or shower.

78. **Keep several sets of clean undergarments in a drawer** in the bathroom so you can change into them after you shower.

79. **Cut your toenails right after you bathe** since they are less brittle and will be easier to cut. A toenail clipper or pair of scissors with short blades works best. However, if your nails are too thick, select a heavy-duty pair of scissors, or consider having your toenails cut by a pedicurist or podiatrist.

80. **After eating, check your mouth for any residual food** and rinse with antibacterial mouthwash. Maintaining good oral hygiene is especially important because the swallowing problems often associated with PD can leave food in your mouth that attracts harmful bacteria.

81. **Use an electric toothbrush** instead of a traditional toothbrush if you have tremors. Brushing your teeth thoroughly with a traditional toothbrush can be difficult. Some electric models have long, easily grasped handles, some are cordless, and some feature dual motion (up and down, side to side). Or try using a toothbrush with an oversized handle, which you can find at most drug stores. Then brush your teeth while sitting down and resting your elbow on the bathroom counter.

82. **Buy dental floss "swords" that look like the letter "C"** at the end of a plastic toothpick with floss stretched tight across the opening. They let you floss with one hand, and are available in drug stores. Or use a WaterPik® to massage your gums and rinse food debris from your

mouth. (It takes some dexterity to use a WaterPik®, so if you have tremors, you might want to stick to rinsing with a sip of water or mouthwash and using dental floss "swords.")

83. **Consider purchasing Toothettes™,** a sponge coated in dried toothpaste, attached to the end of a small stick. They're great for cleaning out the mouth and getting to those areas a toothbrush can't. Dampen it with water or dip it in a little mouthwash to clean out your mouth when brushing isn't convenient.

84. **Use an electric razor if you experience tremors.** Electric razors come in many shapes, some of which are easier to hold than others. Test out how they feel in your hand at the store before you buy one.

85. **Use pump-type containers for lotions and liquid soap.** It's often easier to press down on a pump top than to squeeze a bottle or grasp a bar of soap.

CHOOSING THE RIGHT CLOTHING

86. **Take the hassle out of finding the right clothing.** If shopping for new clothes is overly taxing, call your favorite clothing store and schedule a convenient time when a sales clerk can give you individual attention. In some cities, stores offer personal shopping services. A personal shopper will listen to your clothing needs and specifications and find the appropriate items for you. You can also order from retailers with catalogs or Web sites if you prefer to shop from home.

87. **Replace clothes that are hard to put on with easy-on/easy-off clothes.** You may want to buy clothing one size larger than you normally wear.

88. **Choose satin or nylon tricot sleepwear.** Turning over in bed will be easier because of the slippery surface of satin.

89. **Choose underwear made of nylon** instead of cotton. You will have an easier time pulling slacks and trousers up and down.

90. **Choose clothing that closes in the front if you dress yourself.** If your arms are stiff and you need help dressing, purchase or make shirts that open in the back but look like front-opening shirts.

91. **Choose shirts with multiple colors and patterns** if you tend to spill when eating. Most spills won't show up.

92. **Choose clothing with elastic waistbands or Velcro™ closures** instead of zippers or buttons. Sweatpants that are made of double-knit fabric and have elasticized waistbands are generally easier to put on and take off. Wear pullover tops to eliminate fastening.

DRESSING TIPS

93. **Always dress a weaker limb or your stiffer side first**. To undress, take the garment off the stronger side first.

94. **To remove a shirt or blouse,** unbutton the garment and ease it off your shoulders. Reach behind your back and gently tug the garment off.

95. **Dress in front of a mirror.** It will help you find the sleeves and match up buttons and button-holes. Button garments from the bottom up, so you're less likely to skip a button. Or button the bottom few buttons and put the garment on over your head.

96. **If you're wearing layers,** such as a turtleneck underneath a sweater, put the turtleneck inside the sweater before dressing (don't forget to pull the sleeves through) so you will only have to expend the effort of putting on the garments one time.

👍 **Helping Hands**

97. **If the person with Parkinson's disease is easily confused or upset by change,** try to always dress him or her in the same type of clothing (e.g., sweatpants, a short-sleeved shirt, and a zip-front cardigan).

DRESSING AIDS AND SIMPLE CLOTHING ADAPTATIONS

98. **Use Velcro™ to replace buttons and other fasteners.** Sew an existing buttonhole closed and sew a button on top of it. Then, sew the soft fuzzy side of the Velcro™ on the under side of the closed-up buttonhole. Sew the other piece of Velcro™, the hard side with the small hooks, where the button used to be.

99. **Sew buttons on with elastic thread.** If buttoned cuff openings are too small to pass your fist through, move the buttons to make the opening larger and/or sew the buttons on with elastic thread. The elastic thread will give the rebuttoned cuff opening an extra quarter inch or so.

100. **Make your own zipper pull** by screwing a small cup hook into a dowel. Use it to zip up jackets and dresses. Use a buttonhook. A buttonhook slips through the buttonhole and pulls the button back through it. If your fine motor coordination is impaired, a buttonhook handle is easier to grasp than a small button. Buttonhook handles come in various sizes and finishes (wood, rubber, etc.).

101. **Use a dressing stick so you can dress** while seated (thus reducing your risk of falling). A dressing stick is a long stick with a hook or clamp on the end that you can use to grab items of clothing or accessories and position them on yourself without straining from bending or reaching. You can also use the dressing stick to reach clothing or shoes that have fallen to the floor.

102. **Sew loops of bias tape inside the waistbands** of slacks and trousers. Use the loops to pull pants up and down.

103. **If a waistband is too tight**, extend it by putting a covered ponytail band or rubber band through the buttonhole and wrapping both loops around the button.

HOSIERY AND FOOTWEAR

104. **Choose the right shoes.** If you have a shuffling gait, soft rubber soles make walking more difficult, especially on carpeting, where the soles act like Velcro™ and can cause you to trip. Hard leather soles can be very slippery on linoleum or tile floors.

105. **Use elastic shoelaces** in place of normal laces so you will only have to tie your shoes once. Just slip your shoes on and off.

106. **Have a shoemaker convert your traditional tie- or buckle-close shoes into Velcro™-closing shoes.** Or buy slip-on shoes instead of tie shoes.

107. **Put on your shoes with a long-handled shoehorn** to minimize bending and reaching.

108. **Wear tube socks** because they are easier to put on than socks that are shaped like a foot. Sew loops into the inside of each sock and use the loops to pull on your socks.

109. **Sprinkle cornstarch on the bottom of your feet** and around the heel area to make pulling on nylon stockings or socks easier.

110. **Alter your slacks to accommodate an ankle-foot orthotic (AFO) brace.** If you wear an ankle-foot brace that fits inside a shoe and goes up the calf, it will be easier to dress if you sew a 7-inch zipper into the inside side seam of your slacks.

RESOURCES

111. **To locate clothing that opens in the back,** contact the following companies:

     American Health Care Apparel
     1508 Sullivan Tr.
     Easton, PA 18040
     (800) 252-0584
     (610) 250-0584
     (800) 262-0584 Fax
     http://www.clothesforseniors.com
     info@clothesforseniors.com

     Adrian's Closet
     P.O. Box 65
     San Marcos, CA 92079-0065
     (800) 831-2577
     (714) 364-4380 Fax
     http://www.adrianscloset.com
     adrians@infostations.com

112. **To locate dressing aids, like buttonhooks, zipper pulls, sock aids** contact the following mail-order catalogs:

     Access With Ease
     P.O. Box 1150
     Chino Valley, AZ 86323
     (800) 531-9479
     (520) 636-0292 Fax
     http://shop.store.yahoo.com/capability/index.html
     kmjc@northlink.com

Independent Living aids, inc.
200 Robbins Ln.
Jericho, NY 11753-2341
(800) 537-2118
(516) 752-3135
http://www.independentliving.com
can-do@independentliving.com

Smith & Nephew, Inc.
Rehabilitation Division
N104-W13400 Donges Bay Rd.
P.O. Box 1005
Germantown, WI 53022
(800) 558-8633
(262) 251-7840
(800) 545-7758 Fax
http://www.smith-nephew.com/us/rehab/
rehab.customercare@smith-nephew.com

113. To locate Medi™ compression socks that may relieve painful, swollen feet, consult your doctor. These socks have a stronger compression than the white anti-embolism socks patients often wear in the hospital. You will need a prescription for the socks, which run about $60 per pair. Your insurance might cover part or all of the cost. Putting on the socks requires some strength and practice and you may need assistance. The socks come in navy, black, and flesh tones.

MediUSA L.P.
6481 Franz Warner Pkwy.
Whitsett, N.C. 27377-3000
(800) 633-6334

(866) 223-5234
http://www.mediusa.com
info@mediusa.com

114. **To locate swimsuits that wrap around the body and are extremely easy to put on and take off,** contact:

Suits Me Swimwear
2377 Deltona Blvd.
Spring Hill, FL 34606
(352) 666-1485
http://www.latexfreeswimwear.com
suitsme@star.net

CHAPTER 4

Communicating

Parkinson's disease (PD) can affect communication in many ways. Your ability to speak can diminish because of the disease itself or the medications used to control your symptoms. It is important, though, that you talk for yourself whenever possible. Don't get into the habit of letting others do all the talking for you. Have a discussion with your family and friends about your speech problems, and let them know ways they can help you. Encourage them to ask you to speak louder or ask for a repetition. Try not to be defensive when asked to repeat yourself. Staying calm will make it much easier for you to be heard and understood.

If you are frustrated when a well-meaning family member attempts to fill in words when you pause in a sentence, let him or her know that you just need a little more time to finish, and that you'd appreciate the chance to speak on your own. Set some ground rules about which approaches to communication work for you and which approaches you find less helpful. **The important thing is not to let speech difficulties prevent you from communicating and participating in social activities.**

People with PD sometimes experience the loss of facial expression (masked faces) and have a fixed stare. When this happens many nonverbal cues are lost and there can be misunderstandings and miscommunications. For example: a person with PD may look bored or disapproving, which may not be the case at all. If your facial movements lack expression, make an extra effort to express verbally how you feel and what you are thinking.

Your handwriting may also be affected by PD. Many people find that their writing grows smaller and smaller with each word or letter (micrographia). You might be inclined to give up writing. Don't. Writing is a form of exercise for your hands and arms, and continuing to use those muscles will maintain their condition. Try printing instead of writing in cursive — it can be more legible.

This chapter discusses additional tips for improving your ability to communicate.

SPEAKING TIPS

115. **Take time to organize your thoughts and plan what you are going to say.** If you have trouble remembering or pronouncing a particular word, think of a related word to get your idea across.

116. **Take a breath before you start to speak** and pause every few words, or even between each word. Learn to use your diaphragm when you breathe. (Your stomach will move up and down rather than in and out.) When you breathe cor-

rectly, it will help improve the volume at which you speak and you will have enough air to finish a sentence.

117. **Face your listener.** It will be easier for you to communicate if you can both see each other's faces and if you have each other's full attention. Don't try to carry on a conversation with someone who is in a different room or whom you can't see.

118. **Have conversations in a quiet environment** so you can hear and be heard better. This is especially important if your voice is soft or you have trouble hearing.

119. **Swallow any excess saliva before you attempt to speak.** Or if dry mouth is a problem, keep a water bottle handy so you can take a sip before speaking.

120. **Express yourself in short, concise phrases or sentences.** Use shorter sentences or use only the necessary words to get the message across, even if it's not in complete sentence form.

121. **Exaggerate your pronunciation of words.** Force your tongue, lips, and jaw to work hard as you speak. Enunciate as if your listener is hard of hearing and needs to read your lips. Finish saying the final consonant of a word before beginning the next word. Precise word endings are necessary to determine word meanings (e.g., *them* vs. *then*).

122. **Make a conscious effort to vary your facial expressions** to reflect your mood and the message you're trying to convey. Sometimes

with PD your face is less expressive than it used to be. Integrate the following warm-up activities into your morning or evening washing ritual:

◊ **Massage your facial muscles.**

◊ **Practice in the mirror:** open and close your mouth; alternate smiling and pursing your lips; raise and lower the tip of your tongue, then move your whole tongue from side to side.

◊ **Consciously raise your head to an upright position.** Think about how your head and neck feel.

◊ **Try some verbal warm-ups** like reciting a poem or singing a song.

123. **Close your eyes if you find you are easily distracted while talking.** This will minimize environmental distractions and reduce the pressure you feel in watching the other person waiting for your next word. If you're talking while walking, pause for a moment before closing your eyes (and remember to open your eyes again before you resume walking!).

124. **Use gestures while you talk** to make yourself understood. If you can't think of the word, try pointing to an object you are discussing.

125. **If possible, write what you want to say,** or use a communication board featuring words, the alphabet, or pictures.

126. **When you are frustrated, count to ten.** Allowing stress and frustration to get the better of you will make it even harder for you to communicate.

127. **Use these word-finding tips** if you can't think of the word you want to say:

   ◊ **Say the first sound of the word a few times** until the rest of the word comes to you. Or say a word that rhymes with the one you want. Ask the person you're speaking with to help come up with possibilities until you get to the right word.

   ◊ **Go through the alphabet in your head** until you come to the letter with which the word begins.

   ◊ **Use a category approach:** If you are trying to remember the word for a new item of clothing you bought, think of the words for other kinds of clothing. (Think, "Jacket, slacks, socks, shoes..." until you get to "sweater.")

128 **If you find yourself having unusual difficulty finishing a conversation,** take a break and return to the conversation after you've had a chance to rest a bit.

👍 Helping Hands

129. **Have your hearing and the person with PD hearing checked** to keep your communication from being adversely affected by an inability to hear each other.

👍 Helping Hands

130. **Hold conversations at eye level** and make eye contact during conversation. Sit down if the person with PD is sitting, and assume a

relaxed posture to convey your patience and willingness to listen. Speak clearly and calmly, and allow enough time for a thorough exchange of words. Be patient. Most people with PD who have difficulty speaking have no cognitive difficulty (meaning their minds are just fine); instead, their muscles and nerves are preventing them from speaking as clearly as they did in the past.

☝ Helping Hands

131. **Avoid finishing sentences for someone with PD** unless he asks for your help finding a word or phrase. Reinforce instances of good, intelligible speech. Give feedback such as a nod of the head or a "yes" or "I see" to indicate that you understand what he is saying. However, don't say you understand when you really do not. Repeat any part of the message you did understand and ask for clarification or repetition of the rest. Asking for a repetition of a phrase can result in clearer pronunciation the second time around.

☝ Helping Hands

132. **Ask the person with PD to restate a phrase or sentence using different words** if you cannot understand what was said. If you pretend to understand to save time, misunderstandings can result. In addition, the person with PD may not make as much of an effort to speak clearly if she thinks you understand.

👍 Helping Hands

133. **Ask questions that require yes/no answers.** For example, instead of asking, "What would you like to eat?" ask, "Would you like a turkey sandwich?" Or ask questions that will elicit one-word, or short-phrased responses. Ask, "What kind of meat would you like on your sandwich?" instead of "What do you want for lunch?" Or offer a few choices when you ask a question: "Would you like soup or a sandwich for lunch? Would you like tomato soup or chicken noodle soup?" Use some gentle prompts before beginning a new topic of conversation. Say, for example, "Let's talk about your grandchildren." When you change the subject, use similar cues ("Let's talk about the Super Bowl now").

👍 Helping Hands

134. **Give verbal cues before assisting someone with Parkinson's disease.** If you're going to help someone with an activity, tell the person what you are about to do before you touch him or her. This will reduce your chances of startling the person. For example, before guiding the person to the door, say, "Let's go outside now."

USING TECHNOLOGY TO AID IN SPOKEN COMMUNICATION

135. **Replace hard-to-use telephones** with models that are easier and that can actually enhance your ability to communicate:

◊ **Make a cordless phone even easier to use by adding a headset,** which looks like a headband with a microphone and earphone. Clip the phone to your belt or set it in your lap, and then you can talk hands-free. Headsets cost about $20 and are sold wherever phones are sold.

◊ **Use big button telephones** with large buttons and raised or enlarged numbers and letters. Giant push-button telephone adapters slip easily over the faceplate of most touch tone phones, and they double the size of the numbers to make them easier to see and press.

◊ **Look for telephones with a volume control in the receiver** so you can easily turn the volume up or down during a call.

◊ **Use the special features available on many phones today.** Hands-free speakerphones with built-in speakers and automatic dialing can be fitted with headsets and special on/off switches. Speakerphones and cordless phones often have intercom capabilities, which can be particularly helpful for communicating with people in other rooms of the house.

◊ **Learn how to program your telephone's auto-dial or speed-dial function** to eliminate the need to dial frequently used numbers. Or have a friend or family member program the phone for you and explain how to use the speed-dial features. Write directions down on an index card and keep the card next to the phone, or tape the instructions onto the handset of a cordless phone so they are always there when you need them.

136. **If you have programmed telephone numbers of friends and family into the speed-dial feature of your telephone,** tape small photos of each person next to the button that corresponds to their phone number. Seeing a picture can be a better memory jogger than if just their names or phone numbers are written next to the buttons.

WRITING TIPS

137. **Keep your hand and arm muscles in the habit of writing by taking up drawing or painting.** Not only will you improve the condition of your muscles, but you may find a new artistic talent. If you don't want to start with a blank page, purchase coloring books that have designs, costumes, and nature scenes to color.

138. **Try writing with the hand you don't normally use.** Practicing this can keep both sides of your brain active.

139. **Try printing letters in the opposite direction of what you usually do.** For instance, if you normally write the letter P starting with a straight downward stroke and then lifting your pen to add the half-circle to the top, try starting at the bottom of the P and adding the half-circle in one continuous stroke without lifting the pen. Or make the half-circle first and add the stick later.

140. **Buy pens and pencils with wide grips (at least 1¹/₂ inches (3 cm), because they are easy to grasp and use.** Or make holding a standard pen or pencil easier by trying one of the following:

◊ **Twist a rubber band several times around a pen or pencil.** Roll it into position where your fingers rest. The rubber band will widen the barrel and help you keep your grip.

◊ **Slip a 2-inch piece of rubber tubing over the barrel of a pen or pencil** to make the grip easier to use.

◊ **Use pen or pencil grips.** These grips are small, cylindrical pieces of rubber with a hole in the center. The pen or pencil fits through the hole and you adjust the rubber grip until it is in a comfortable writing position. It stays in place until you move it or take it off. These devices can be found at office or school supply stores.

141. **Bring along several preprinted, self-adhesive address labels** (with your name and address) when you attend conventions, forums, store openings, or any other place you might need to fill out forms. Instead of writing all your information on the form, use your address labels when you want to sign up, register for prizes, or send away for information. You can also purchase a rubber stamp with your address or signature on it.

KEEPING THE LINES
OF COMMUNICATION OPEN

142. **Use the computer to communicate when speaking or writing is too difficult.** Going online and communicating with others will help keep your mind active. Using e-mail can

be a wonderful way to keep in touch with family and friends.

👍 Helping Hands

143. **Encourage friends and relatives to each choose a specific time each day or each week to call.** Having short (2- or 3-minute) conversations on a regular basis can go a long way toward helping the person feel included and loved especially if he or she can't get out socially.

👍 Helping Hands

144. **If someone you care for is unable to leave the home for special events such as reunions and weddings,** use a video camera to document the event. Have people at the event record special greetings for the person who was unable to make it. If you move to a new home and your loved one cannot visit, make home videos of your new house, the neighborhood, the kids' school, soccer field, library, etc. When you deliver the video, give a running narration of the scenes shown on the screen. It can be a great way to spend time together and keep the person involved in your life.

👍 Helping Hands

145. **Use your camcorder to create a video "card" for someone who can't get out to visit family and friends.** Record well wishes and other greetings, and also take footage of some of the person's favorite places. This unique document will spark

fond memories and show the person that he or she is remembered.

RESOURCES

146. **For consumer information about firms handling specialized equipment and the names of associations and support groups,** contact your local library reference desk.

147. **Speech-to-Speech Relay (or Telecommunications Relay Service)** is a federally mandated service for people whose speech may be difficult to understand because of a medical condition, or because they use a voice synthesizer, voice enhancer, or electrolarynx. The service helps remove the communication barriers that people with speech disorders face when they are doing something as basic as ordering a pizza or making a doctor's appointment. The person with the speech disability calls the telecommunications relay system in his or her state, and a specially trained communication assistant (CA) takes down the number that the person with the speech disability wants to call. To make a doctor's appointment, for example, the CA calls the doctor's appointment desk on the phone, listens to the person with the speech disability and repeats the message word-for-word to the doctor's receptionist. Communication continues with the CA acting as the voice of the person with the speech disorder.

    The telecommunications relay system also facilitates calls between people who use a standard phone and those who use a TTY (or text telephone) due to hearing impairments. As of

March 1, 2001 all states are required to provide Speech-to-Speech/Telecommunication Relay Services 24 hours a day, seven days a week. Check the "Rights and Responsibilities" pages in the beginning of your local telephone book, or call your state's Department of Administration for details. For additional information on Speech-to-Speech Relay, visit www.stsnews.com

148. **Speech amplifiers** can be helpful to people with PD who have a weak voice, throat, or chest muscles, partially paralyzed vocal cords, or diminished lung capacity. Speech amplifiers are like portable public address systems, and they can improve one-on-one and group communication by allowing the speaker to use his or her normal tone, but amplifying it so that listeners can hear the voice better. Some amplifiers are pocket size, and some have handheld or headset microphones. The following companies sell a variety of speech amplifying products:

Amplivox Sound Systems
3149 MacArthur Blvd.
Northbrook , IL 60062
(847) 498-9000
(847) 498-6691 Fax
http://www.ampli.com
info@ampli.com

Luminaud, Inc.
8688 Tyler Blvd.
Mentor, OH 44060
(800) 255-3408
(440) 255-9082
(440) 255-2250 Fax
http://www.luminaud.com
info@luminaud.com

Park Surgical Co., Inc.
5001 New Utrecht Ave.
Brooklyn, NY 11219
(800) 633-7878
(718) 436-9200
http://www.parksurgical.com
ParkSurgic@aol.com

Chapter 5

Managing Mealtime Madness

The kitchen is often the busiest room in the house. It becomes a hotbed of activity when you're preparing and eating meals. The chapter on General Home Accessibility shares kitchen organization tips. This chapter will help you plan, make, and serve meals so you can streamline the process and make tasks easier.

Begin by building more time into your schedule to prepare and eat meals. Make the kitchen or dining room a calm, low-stress environment by playing soft, relaxing music while you cook and eat.

Do as much planning and preparation as possible while seated at the kitchen table or at a stool pulled up to a countertop. If your energy or medication's effectiveness waxes and wanes, prepare meals when your energy level is high, and reheat it and serve after you've had a chance to rest. When eating, sit close to the table and place all food and utensils within easy reach.

IN THE KITCHEN

Meal Planning and Preparation

149. **Choose a grocery store that will not defeat you before you begin.** When deciding on a store, take into account not only prices and location but also layout and facilities, including restrooms. Is the store accessible? Are the doors easy to manage? Are the floors clear of debris and obstacles?

150. **Ask if your neighborhood grocery store has a home delivery service** if getting out to shop for groceries is a problem. Some stores will charge a flat fee, while others will require a minimum order. Delivery areas vary and so does how far in advance you must call to place your order. Large chain stores or warehouse-type grocery stores rarely deliver but they often have the names and phone numbers of delivery services that do. Or order your groceries from an online service (see the Resources section at the end of this chapter).

151. **If you don't want to walk unassisted through a slippery parking lot,** some grocery stores will send a bagger or stock person to help you get from your car to the store door and back again. Other stores may allow you to pull up to the front door and have an employee park your car. These services are available to regular customers who have made arrangements in advance. Another option is to park next to the area where shopping carts are kept outside. Pushing a shopping cart can improve your stability when walking through the parking lot and store.

152. **Ask the bagger to not fill your bags too full.** Spread out the items into more, but lighter-weight, bags. Ask that all frozen or perishable foods be put into one bag. Then when you arrive home you only need to empty one bag immediately, and the others can wait.

153. **To make grocery shopping faster and more efficient,** create a diagram of the store and list the food categories for each aisle. Then make a master list on your computer of items you buy. Before you go to the store, print out a list and circle each item you need. This method is especially helpful if you send a friend to do your grocery shopping — then there is no question about what brand and what size of a particular item you want.

154. **Use a wagon (like a Radio Flyer™) or a wheeled wire cart to move groceries from the car to the house.**

👍 **Helping Hands**

155. **Encourage the person with PD to be involved in activities like sorting things** — putting away groceries, setting the table and putting away clean silverware and dishes. If items are not put in the proper spot, quietly move them to where they belong.

156. **To open a jar if your hands are weak,** improve your grip by putting on a rubber glove, by winding a thick rubber band twice around the lid, or by using a 5" x 5", thin, waffle-grid rubber sheet, available where kitchen gadgets are sold.

These rubberized sheets make untwisting caps and lids easier. Other jar openers (that attach to the underside of a cabinet) are also available.

157. **Use a rocker knife instead of a traditional straight knife.** You can get a seesaw motion going with the rocker knife and use less energy than required with a straight knife.

158. **Keep an extra pair of pliers in the kitchen.** Use them to peel away the plastic seal from a jar of peanut butter, to pull the tab on a container of cream cheese, and to grab the sealer strip from a can of frozen orange juice or a gallon of milk.

159. **Purchase jelly in plastic squeeze bottles** so spreading it on sandwiches is easier.

160. **If you have tremors, prepare finger foods that don't require use of a knife and fork.** Purchase cheese cubes, precut chicken strips, and cocktail-sized hot dogs just to name a few. In the produce section of the grocery store, you'll find cut up fruits and vegetables. While they sometimes cost more than the uncut variety, the time and energy you save can be worth every penny.

Making and/or Using Simple Adaptive Devices at Mealtimes

161. **If grasping and holding onto silverware is difficult,** use modeling clay to build up the handles. Or take foam tubing, which comes in a variety of thicknesses, and build up the handles on utensils. Another solution is to purchase stainless steel flatware with big bamboo or plastic handles that are easier to grip. Some

specialty catalogs and medical supply stores sell inexpensive utensils specially designed for easy use. (Using weighted, built-up utensils may also help decrease tremors while eating.)

162. **Use a glass or metal pie pan instead of a regular plate** if you have trouble keeping food from sliding off the plate. Use a plate guard or a pasta bowl with high sides because it will be easier to get food onto the spoon or fork. Plate guards can be attached to plates to provide a rim on one side. Use your fork to push food against the guard, where food will fall onto the fork. Plate guards also help reduce spills.

163. **Place Dycem™ rubber pads or Rubbermaid™ mats underneath plates, cups, and serving dishes** to keep them from sliding.

164. **Make handling a drinking glass easier if you have hand tremors or a weakened grip:**

    ◊ **Fill glasses half-full.**

    ◊ **Wind several thick rubber bands around the glass.**

    ◊ **Drink from a plastic water bottle (or sports bottle)** instead of a glass. The small opening at the top prevents beverages from sloshing out, and when sealed, the cap prevents spills if the bottle is accidentally bumped.

    ◊ **Use a flexible plastic drinking straw instead of drinking directly out of a glass.** To better hold a straw in place, find a lid of a plastic container (the same diameter as your glass), punch a hole in the lid, and insert a straw into the hole. You'll find that the straw does not slide around in the glass.

◊ **Use a child's cup with a built-in straw for drinking.** The Tommee Tippee™ cup is made of unbreakable plastic and has a spout and a see-through cover. The curved base is weighted to prevent spilling.

◊ **Drink from a cup or mug that has two handles.**

EATING AND DRINKING TIPS FOR PEOPLE WITH SWALLOWING DIFFICULTIES

Swallowing is a very complex process, and difficulties in chewing or swallowing (dysphagia) can cause additional health problems. It is estimated that 50% of people with PD will experience dysphagia at some time during the course of their illness.

If you experience difficulty swallowing, ask your doctor for a referral to a speech/language pathologist (SLP), along with a prescription for "swallowing evaluation and therapy." A swallowing study and a video fluoroscopic evaluation by a specially trained SLP can best diagnose exactly what part of the swallowing process is causing you problems, and recommend a treatment program for you. You and the people who help you will learn important tips that can help keep you healthy.

One important consideration affecting swallowing ease may be when you take your medication. Consult with your physician on how to time your medications to facilitate swallowing, and experiment with what works best for you.

To reduce swallowing difficulties

165. **Plan a regular mealtime schedule.** Give yourself at least twice the time it usually takes to eat the meal. Don't allow yourself to feel hurried, because stress can exacerbate symptoms and make swallowing even more difficult. Minimize mealtime distractions by turning off the television and radio and keeping conversation to a minimum.

     If you find that you fatigue too much when eating a whole meal, plan 5 or 6 smaller meals during the day or snack throughout the day. If chewing is too difficult, but your swallowing is good, drink a food supplement such as Ensure™, Boost™, or Carnation Instant Breakfast™ to supplement your diet. Check with your doctor to make sure that the protein content of those drinks doesn't interfere with the absorption of your medications.

166. **Suck on a few crushed ice cubes about 20 minutes before mealtime** to reduce any swelling in your throat. Or eat something very cold and sour like lemon or lime sherbet before you begin to eat. This may help to improve saliva production for people with dry mouth. It may also stimulate the muscles necessary for swallowing and reduce tongue delay. Although not proven, it may be helpful to eat spoonfuls of the cold, sour food periodically during the meal to continue improved swallowing and to help clear the mouth and throat of food particles.

167. **Sit in an upright position with both feet on the floor,** and stay upright for at least 30

minutes after a meal. Reclining or lying flat while eating can cause food to remain in the esophagus or to back up into it. If you have frequent heartburn, it is important to consult with a good gastroenterologist. Frequent bouts of heartburn can damage the esophagus. In rare cases, food can be refluxed all the way up and into the throat. The major danger when that happens is that some of the refluxed material could get into the airway and down into the lungs. When foreign material gets into the lungs, it can cause pneumonia.

168. **Keep your chin pointed down as you chew and swallow.** In addition, gently touching or massaging the front of the throat right before or during eating may help stimulate swallowing.

169. **Concentrate on each step of the swallowing process.** Make sure you have enough saliva or moisture in your mouth to get the food into your esophagus. Do not try to eat if you are too fatigued to concentrate on chewing and swallowing.

170. **Take bite-sized portions** (about one-half spoonful) of food. Chew deliberately. Swallow each bite completely before you take another. Chew hard with the food on one side of the mouth, and then move the food to the other side and chew hard some more. Take comfortable sips of liquids to reduce the risk of aspiration. If swallowing liquids at the same time as solid foods is difficult, stick to one substance at a time before you try to swallow another.

171. **If you have a cough that you can't stop,** try eating a spoonful of applesauce. Its cool, smooth texture can help soothe your irritated throat. Applesauce now comes in single-serving cups so you can carry one with you for instant relief.

     However, if your cough persists, food may have gone down into your airway. A cough is your body's natural protective mechanism for getting rid of foreign material in the airway. The signs of silent aspiration (food particles that go into the airway, but you do not feel them) may be respiratory problems, fever, chest noises, and then pneumonia. Consult a doctor immediately if you experience any of these symptoms.

172. **If you feel that you are choking while swallowing,** close your mouth, breathe through your nose, and calm down. Taking that one breath will give you enough air to help avoid panic and will help you breathe normally. Ask family members and helpers to learn the Heimlich maneuver in case you choke while trying to swallow. A doctor or other healthcare professional can demonstrate and teach the procedure.

Tips If Drooling Is a Problem

173. **When drooling is a problem, chew gum.** It helps remind you to swallow more often.

174. **Make it a deliberate habit to try to swallow your saliva regularly** to reduce its accumulation in your mouth. Close your lips firmly, move the saliva to the back of your throat, and swallow. Swallow any excess saliva before you attempt to speak.

Food consistency and texture

175. **The texture of food becomes more important** when you can taste only sweet, sour, or salt. See which textures work better for you. However, if you have trouble swallowing, be sure to have a swallowing study done, which can tell you if thickened liquids might help and how to experiment with various degrees of thickness.

176. **Swallowing can be easier if you stick with foods of a soft, even consistency.** An example would be creamy, whipped mashed potatoes (not lumpy and dry, on the one hand, and not thin and runny, on the other, but smooth and somewhat viscous like sour cream).

177. **Avoid foods that easily pose a choking hazard:**

    ◊ **Steak** is the number one thing people choke on. Eat ground steak instead.

    ◊ **Dry foods that break into small pieces** like seeds, nuts, or baked goods.

    ◊ **Foods that irritate your throat** (such as vinegar) or cause you to choke (potato chips, etc.).

178. **Stick with foods that are easy to swallow:**

    ◊ **Baby foods and cereals.** Baby foods have a smooth, easy-to-swallow consistency.

    ◊ **Strained, thickened soups.** Puree a favorite soup in a food processor or blender to remove chunks. Then, thicken the soup with mashed potatoes (or strained, mashed peas, beans, lentils, or chickpeas), blend, and serve.

◊ **Strained, thickened fruits.** Use a food processor to combine your favorite fruits with cottage cheese, cream cheese, or yogurt. Strain off excess liquid, blend until desired consistency is reached, and then serve.

◊ **Yogurt.** Buy the smooth or blended variety, or puree the fruit-on-the-bottom variety in a blender until smooth.

◊ **Thick puddings.**

◊ **Soft bread with crusts removed.** Take your time with bread. Eat one small piece at a time. Suck on it until it is soaked in saliva, and swallow it with one big gulp.

◊ **Canned liquid diets.** Some of these may be too thin, so you can thicken them with cornstarch. Also, relying solely on liquid diets can result in low blood albumin, so you might want to add dried egg white powder to the liquid if you plan to use liquid diets for an extended period.

◊ **Fruit nectars.** Thicker than most juices, nectars are less likely to be aspirated when swallowed. Look for apricot, pear, mango, and banana nectar in the ethnic or specialty aisle of your supermarket. Tomato juice is another thicker beverage that can be easier to swallow.

◊ **Thick spreads like hummus or cream cheese.** Serve on soft, crustless bread or eat as a snack with a spoon.

◊ **Mashed avocado or banana.**

179. **Try variations on your favorite food and drinks** to make them easier to swallow. For instance, if you find regular orange juice irritating to your throat, try orange juice with pulp, or the low-acidity kind.

Swallowing Pills and Vitamins

180. **Some pills can be difficult to swallow,** so ask your doctor or pharmacist if your medication will retain its potency if it is ground up and combined with food. If your doctor advises against grinding up your pills, try swallowing the pill with fruit nectar instead of water. Or swallow it along with a spoonful of applesauce or honey, or try coating the pill with a little butter or pudding.

181. **Put the pill into your mouth, tilt your chin down, look down into the bottom of your glass of water, and swallow.** Continue to look down during the entire swallowing process. Some people find that this works much better than tilting your head backwards when swallowing a pill.

RESOURCES

182. **Online grocery stores are a convenient way to shop.** You can periodically place your order over the Internet to avoid going out in inclement weather or you can schedule regular grocery delivery of your favorite foods. Unfortunately, this type of service only covers certain areas of the country. Continue to check these Web sites for changes in their delivery areas. Also, check your local grocery

stores to see if they offer online grocery shopping or home delivery.

◊ www.peapod.com

◊ www.netgrocer.com

183. **Thickeners can make liquids and prepared foods easier to swallow.** Diamond Crystal brand (http://www.diamondcrystal.com) makes a product called Thicken Right® Instant Food Thickener, which can be mixed with liquids and prepared foods to thicken them to whatever consistency you desire. Order their products from any of the following distributors:

D.C. Distributors, Inc.
P.O. Box 224
Amherst, NY 14226
(800) 827-6763
(716) 825-5834
http://www.dcdistributors.com
dc@dcdistributors.com

Med-Diet Laboratories
3600 Holly Ln., Ste. 80
Plymouth, MN 55447
(800) MED-DIET
(800) 633-3438
(763) 550-2022 Fax
http://www.med-diet.com
meddiet@med-diet.com

Bruce Medical
411 Waverly Oaks Rd., Ste. 154
Waltham, MA 02452

(800) 225-8446
(781) 894-9519 Fax
http://www.brucemedical.com
sales@brucemedical.com

184. **"Swallowing Safely, Swallowing Nutritiously: A Manual for the Swallowing Impaired"** written by Maxine Dereiko, a Registered, Licensed Dietitian and Patricia Stout MS, CCC and "Recipes for Easy Chewing and Safe Swallowing" by Dereiko and Elaine Teutsch, R.N., MS offer help to people with moderate to severe swallowing problems. $15 plus $3.50 for shipping and handling. Allow 4-6 weeks for delivery.

Dereiko-Teutsch & Associates
P.O. Box 8366
Portland, OR 97207
(503) 241-8077
(503) 241-1490 Fax
http://www.dereiko.com

185. **There are many adaptive devices to make meal preparation, eating, and drinking easier.** Contact the following companies for a catalog:

Sammons-Preston, Inc. (Enrichments)
A Subsidiary of Bissell Health Care Corp.)
P.O. Box 5071
Bollingbrook, IL 60440
(800) 323-5547
(800) 547-4333 Fax
http://www.sammonspreston.com
sp@sammonspreston.com

Easy Street
8 Spring Brook Road
Foxboro, MA 02035
(800) 959-EASY
http:www.easystreetco.com
support@easystreetco.com

Maxi Aids, Inc.
42 Executive Blvd.
Farmingdale, NY 11735
(800) 522-6294
(631) 752-0521
(631) 752-0738 TTY
(631) 752-0689 Fax
http://www.maxiaids.com
sales@maxiaids.com

Smith & Nephew Inc. Rehab
P.O. Box 1005
Germantown, WI 53022-8205
(800) 558-8633
(800) 545-7758 Fax
http://www.smith-nephew.com

CHAPTER 6

Empowering Yourself

L ife is about choices. You may not have total control over your Parkinson's disease (PD), but you *do* have control about how you let it affect your life. Staying active and involved is possible with effort and determination.

Keep moving. Eliminate distractions and tell your family and friends that you may not be able to carry on a conversation when you are walking. If crowds or long distance walking is involved, use a cane or walker for stability. Pushing a baby stroller or shopping cart can also help you maintain balance. Using a wheelchair may also be an option, especially at museums, sidewalk art shows, and amusement parks. Choose to make the necessary compromises and adjustments so you can stay involved in family and community activities.

Another way to stay active and involved is to continue doing the quiet leisure activities you enjoy. If the effects of PD or your medications make your favorite hobby difficult to pursue, try a variation on your hobby or learn a new craft. Keep your mind and your hands active by doing jigsaw puzzles, taking up painting or woodworking, or playing a musical instrument. Take a class so you can learn along with others and meet new people who share your interests. You'll socialize and learn something at the same time. If you have a skill that you haven't used in a while, pick up a beginner's book at the library and refresh your memory with introductory lessons. You'll be surprised at how quickly you can relearn a skill you thought you'd forgotten. Don't be hard on yourself if it takes you a while to master a new craft, though. Everybody has a learning curve. Don't let initial frustrations discourage you from keeping at it.

Some people who have PD have trouble with concentration, memory, or communication problems. If you feel these abilities have been affected, there is help. Discuss your concerns with your doctor and ask to see a psychologist who will be able to help you identify exactly what cognitive deficits you might be experiencing, and help you develop plans to keep effectively on track.

Here are some other tips to get you moving, involved, and enjoying the fun things in life.

MOBILITY AND EXERCISE

Walking

185. **Walking with someone can be better than using a walker.** Hold onto the arm of someone else while walking, and say out loud together, "Left, right, left, right, left, right." This might help you concentrate on your movements. Your physical therapist (PT) can help determine when using a walker is safer.

186. **When walking, bring your toes up with every step you take.** If you tend to shuffle, follow these steps:

   ◊ **Stop walking.**

   ◊ **Make sure your feet are about eight inches apart.**

   ◊ **Stand up as straight as you can.**

   ◊ **Think about taking a large step.**

   ◊ **Take a step by bringing one foot up high,** as in a marching fashion.

   ◊ **Lift your toes up and place your heel down first.**

   ◊ **Roll onto the ball of your foot and toes.**

   ◊ **Repeat this process with the other foot.**

   ◊ **Swing your opposite arm forward when taking a step.** This will improve the rhythm of your walking and your appearance. Swinging your arms freely while walking, shifts body weight from your legs, lessens fatigue, and it helps loosen your arms and shoulders.

187. **If you drag your foot, see an orthopedic specialist.** Untreated, your foot dragging will become worse and you will trip yourself. Your orthopedist can make arrangements for you to get an AFO (ankle-foot orthotic) brace. If stumbling persists, see your neurologist.

189. **When you want to turn, don't pivot on one foot by crossing your legs.** Walk into your turn. Walk around in a semicircle with your feet apart.

190. **Try marking your floors with a grid of 18-inch squares of colored electrical tape.** Some people with PD find that it is easier to walk in the squares of tile flooring.

👍 **Helping Hands**

191. **Never grab an arm or try to help a person without asking first if they would like your help.** Let the person with PD tell you how to help him or her. Remember, you are supplying balance control, not physical support. Don't try to pull the person along or lift him or her.

👍 **Helping Hands**

192. **Before you start walking, count down from the number five to the number one.** On one, begin walking. Let the person whom you are assisting set the pace. When appropriate, announce upcoming changes in the terrain ("There's a step down.")

👍 **Helping Hands**

193. **To help a person with PD walk, stand in front of him and hold his hands.** When you walk backwards, gently guide them forward. Give verbal cues like "Let's walk now."

👍 **Helping Hands**

194. **If the person with PD wears bifocals, he or she may need extra help when using stairs.** Going down stairs is often more difficult than walking up. When we go upstairs, we usually look

through the top (or long-distance range) part of the lens, but when we go downstairs, we look down (through the near-distance or reading part of the lens). Looking down, our feet aren't close enough for our eyes to focus on through the reading part of the bifocal. No matter which direction you are going — up or down stairs — watch carefully.

👍 Helping Hands

195. **When assisting someone walking up or down stairs, do not take more than one stair at a time.** Let the person you are assisting hold onto a handrail, if one is available. Make sure he or she places each foot completely on each stair. When going up stairs, have the person lead with the stronger foot. When going down stairs, have the person lead with the weaker foot. Stand in front of the person when descending stairs, and behind the person when ascending the stairs.

Tremors

196. **If you have a tremor, wait until it stops to resume your movement.** Tremors often decrease when you stretch your hands and arms out in front of you.

197. **If a resting tremor interferes with activities involving your hands,** press the affected elbow against your body to stabilize the upper arm, and then perform the desired movement as quickly as you can.

198. **Wear exercise weights around your wrist** (known as wrist weights) to help stabilize

and reduce the frequency and duration of tremors.

Freezing

199. **To get "unstuck" from a freeze that may occur when you approach narrow spaces,** try these tips:

    ◊ **Don't try to take any steps.**

    ◊ **Place your heels on the floor.**

    ◊ **Straighten yourself into an upright posture.** Don't lean backwards or forwards.

    ◊ **Gently rock side to side.**

    ◊ **Take a few marching steps in place.**

    ◊ **Start taking steps forward by placing your heels down first.**

    ◊ **Keep your feet about eight inches apart and correct your posture as you go.**

200. **If you freeze when walking,** try these tips:

    ◊ **Very carefully walk backwards or sideways.**

    ◊ **Count from one to ten, or count by twos to twenty, with the idea in mind that you'll walk when you reach the last number.**

    ◊ **Ask your helper to gently rock back and forth with you to get you moving.**

    ◊ **Try dancing instead of walking.** Whistling or singing may also help you overcome freezing.

    ◊ **Focusing on the beam of a flashlight or laser pointer may break a frozen gait.** Use a credit card-type flashlight instead of a bulky wand-style flashlight. The credit

card varieties are lightweight and convenient, and are activated with a gentle
squeeze. Some come with a key chain
attached, which you can hang from a
bedpost, wheelchair, or walker.

◊ **Try lifting just your toes.**

◊ **Have someone drop pieces of a tissue on
floor like stepping stones and use them to
break your freeze.**

201. **Using a cane can help with freezing.** If you use
a cane with a small golf club-type protrusion at
the bottom, it can make walking easier because
it tricks your mind into thinking you're stepping over something.

202. **Take a collapsible cane with you when you
walk.** When you freeze, assemble the cane and
gently kick the end near the floor.

203. **When you can't walk a step forward,** take a
small step *back*, then rock forward and go.
When you can't turn left, take a small step *right*,
then rock to your left foot and go.

☝ **Helping Hands**

204. **When the person with PD gets stuck in a
freeze,** try taking his or her hands in yours (as
you face him or her) and gently pumping your
hands up and down in an alternating motion.

Standing up, sitting down

205. **If you have trouble standing up from a seated
position,** try these techniques:

◊ **Put your hands on the armrests, rock back and forth, and count.**

◊ **Ask someone to stand in front of you and wiggle or dance.**

◊ **Ask someone to lift up your thigh and bring your foot one step forward.** Quickly, have them do the same thing with the other leg. Then try to stand up.

◊ **Bring your buttocks close to the edge of the chair.** Keep your feet at least eight inches apart, with one foot slightly in front of the other. Rock your trunk quickly back and forth a few times to build up momentum. On your last rock forward, bring your shoulders forward, just past your knees, and push down with your hands on the arms of the chair or the cushion while you straighten up to a standing position.

Mobility devices

206. **Take a cane to help stabilize your walking when visiting unfamiliar places.** People will usually try to be more careful not to bump into you when they see a cane.

207. **If you use a cane and must go out in icy weather,** screw into the bottom of your cane a removable ice gripper tip. Or use a ski pole instead of a cane when walking on icy sidewalks.

208. **If you use a cane in winter and have difficulty gripping the cane handle while wearing mittens or gloves,** knit or crochet a small sleeve to fit snugly over the handle. The woolen glove

and the woolen cover will work together to keep the handle from slipping.

209. **Use a walking stick that resembles a shepherd's staff if you have trouble walking with a traditional cane** but need support when you walk. Your elbow is bent at a 90-degree angle and the staff is in front of you. The staff also helps you stand up straighter when your back muscles are weak. To see if walking with a staff helps you, get a broom or mop and cut the handle off. Put a rubber crutch protector on the end that touches the floor.

210. **Consider using a wheeled walker.** Models are available with wheels and brakes, a seat in the middle for you to rest, and a basket above the wheels to put loose items in. You can hang a tote bag or a wicker bicycle basket from the top to keep important items handy, like your cordless telephone, a box of tissues, a pen, and a small notebook. Have a shoemaker make two special buckle straps for you to thread through the basket and attach to your walker (or to the handlebars of your three-wheeled scooter, if you use one).

211. **Adapt a traditional walker for easier use:** Put three-inch wheels on the front legs and tennis balls on the back legs of a walker, especially if you have thick or looped carpeting.

Mobility resources

212. **The Phil-E-Slide is an ergonomically designed patient lift system that may be**

helpful to caregivers and to people who are unable to move themselves. The system has been in use in England's healthcare facilities since 1992, when a "minimal" or "no-lift" policy was instituted in an effort to reduce risk of personal injury to caregivers. The Phil-E-Slide system is made of ultra-low friction material that improves comfort and independence by enabling a person to transfer with significantly less discomfort and by giving him the ability to assist in the transfer process. The system is easy to carry, transport, use, and clean, and comes with an 18-month guarantee.

Phil-E-Slide
101 Boardman Rd.
Poughkeepsie, NY 12603-4244
(888) 675-4338
(914) 483-9660
(914) 483-0653 Fax
http://www.phil-e-slide.com.

213. **Amigo Mobility International, Inc. produces three-wheeled scooters that are narrower than most conventional wheelchairs and other scooters, making them easier to get through doorways.** Amigo scooters are ideal for people with walking difficulties that are brought on by various conditions, including arthritis, postpolio syndrome, chronic fatigue, multiple sclerosis, muscular dystrophy, amputations, or heart disease. The Amigo helps to save energy and transport people over longer distances. It's perfect for getting around the house or the store, taking a trip around the block, or traveling on

vacation. The Amigo can be dismantled into three separate pieces for easy storage in the trunk of most cars.

Amigo Mobility International, Inc.
6693 Dixie Highway
Bridgeport, MI 48722
(800) MY-AMIGO
(800) 692-6446
(989) 777-8184 Fax
http://www.myamigo.com
info@myamigo.com

214. **Bruno Independent Living Aids, Inc. produces accessibility and mobility products for people with disabilities.** These products include battery powered three- and four-wheeled scooters; automobile, truck, and van lifts to transport scooters, wheelchairs, and power chairs; and stair lifts that allow access to upper and lower levels of buildings.

Bruno Independent Living Aids, Inc.
1780 Executive Dr.
P.O. Box 84
Oconomowoc, WI 53066
(800) 882-8183
(262) 567-4990
(262) 953-5501 Fax
http://www.bruno.com

215. **SpinLife.com is an Internet-based retailer that features a wide selection of wheelchairs, scooters, and accessories at guaranteed low prices.**

SpinLife.com
1108 City Park Ave., Ste. 201
Columbus, OH 43206
(800) 850-0335
(614) 449-8123
(888) 873-6543 Fax
http://www.spinlife.com
customerservice@spinlife.com

216. **Natural Access features Landeez all-terrain and beach wheelchairs.**

Natural Access
P.O. Box 5729
Santa Monica, CA 90409-5729
(800) 411-7789
(310) 392-9864
http://www.natural-access.com/

217. **Service dogs, similar to leader dogs for the blind, can help people with Parkinson's disease and other serious mobility problems.** Service dogs can be trained to assist a person with balance, help get him or her out of a freeze, and assist if the person falls. The dogs have been shown to significantly reduce people's tendency to fall, and they provide a source of unconditional affection that can be greatly beneficial to anyone, regardless of impairment.

Independence Dogs, Inc.
146 State Line Rd.
Chadds Ford, PA 19317
(610) 358-2723
http://www.independencedogs.org
idi@independencedogs.org

LEISURE AND RECREATIONAL ACTIVITIES

Reading

218. Use a ruler or piece of paper as a guide to help your eyes track the lines on the page you are reading.

219. Use the eraser on a pencil or a rubber fingertip (like those used by secretaries and bookkeepers) to turn pages in a book.

220. **Purchase a full-page sheet magnifier** made of wafer-thin plastic that magnifies an entire page at one time. Or use a hand held magnifier to help you look up telephone numbers, scan maps, examine floor plans, read operating instructions or stock market reports, handle hobby & needlecraft projects, etc. Lighted magnifiers are also available from book, craft, or home health stores.

221. **If you listen to audio books, position the tape recorder and stand/table in a convenient position that you can reach.** Then, mark the location of the stand on the floor with masking tape so anyone can easily set up the audio books for you.

Watching television

222. **Purchase or make a bedside pocket to hold eyeglasses, flashlight, pencil, crossword puzzle book, etc.** where half of the material fits between the mattress and the box spring and half the material hangs down the side of the bed and has pockets that holds your glasses, pencil, book etc. Or create your own saddlebag style holder for

your TV and VCR remote control devices, which rests on the arm of your favorite chair. Select two hand towels that fit with your decor and room colors and sew them together at one end making one long piece. Then, fold up each end creating pockets to hold your remotes. If possible divide one of the pockets in half and use it to hold a pencil and note pad. You may also want to secure your holder to the arm of your couch or chair with a few stitches or Velcro™.

223. **Purchase a universal remote control and program it to operate both the VCR and the TV.** Universal remotes cost less than $20 and can be used in the home and elsewhere to operate the TV, VCR, stereo, and DVD player.

224. **Use a large-button adapter** if you have trouble with fine motor movements and are unable to press the buttons on a traditional remote control. The remote sits in an attractive holder and large keys fit over and snap onto the small remote buttons. You can then press the buttons with your fist or the side of your hand. Another device, the Big 'N Easy Wireless TV Remote Control, replaces the remote entirely. A 12-inch × 15-inch plastic console contains large 2-inch buttons that perform all the basic functions of your remote. The buttons are easy to see and push with the palm of your hand. Its infrared wireless technology is compatible with most remote control TVs and cable boxes.

225. **Take a plain adhesive-backed label and write the cable channels and their numbers on it.** Then put the label on the back of your remote

control so you don't have to remember all the numbers or page through a *TV Guide* whenever you want to watch.

Playing games

226. **Try doing crossword puzzles or playing games like Scrabble™, Scattergories™, and Taboo™ to** help exercise your ability to remember words. Playing Trivial Pursuit™ is another great way to keep your memory in shape. If you enjoy watching game shows on television, play along at home. Say the answers aloud while watching *Wheel of Fortune, Jeopardy!,* or *Who Wants to be a Millionaire.*

227. **Use jumbo playing cards,** available at most drug stores or toy stores, which are easier to use than regular cards. To make holding cards easier, take an old shoebox, remove the top, and put the bottom of the box inside the cover. The space between the cover and the side of the shoebox holds the cards nicely.

Leisure and recreation resources

228. **The National Library Service for the Blind and Physically Handicapped (NLS).** More than 159,000 biographies, best sellers, classics, poetry, mysteries, how-to, and other books, as well as 70 popular magazines, are recorded on cassette tapes. A special tape recorder is needed to play the tapes. These recorders, as well as accessories like headphones, remote control units, and amplifiers are available from the Talking Books program. All items and services connected with this program are free. Even the postage on the books is paid. You are eligible

for Talking Books if you meet any of the following criteria:

◊ **You are unable to read standard print without aids or devices other than glasses or contact lenses.**

◊ **You have a visual acuity of less than 20/200 or a visual field of 20 degrees or less with correction.**

◊ **You are unable to hold a book or turn a page.**

◊ **You have a temporary loss of vision or use of your hands.**

◊ **You have a medically documented reading disability.**

To obtain more information or to sign up for this state and federally funded program, contact your local library. Or call the National Library Service for the Blind and Physically Handicapped at (800) 424-9100. The operator will forward your request to the regional library nearest you.

229. **Large button adapters for TV/VCR remote controls can be obtained from the following companies:**

Enrichments for Better Living
Sammons Preston
(An AbilityOne Corporation)
4 Sammons Ct.
Bolingbrook, IL 60440
(800) 323-5547
(800) 547-4333 Fax
http://www.sammonspreston.com
sp@sammonspreston.com

Smith & Nephew, Inc.
Rehabilitation Division
N104-W13400 Donges Bay Rd.
P.O. Box 1005
Germantown, WI 53022
(800) 558-8633
(262) 251-7840
(800) 545-7758 Fax
http://www.smith-nephew.com/us/rehab/
rehab.customercare@smith-nephew.com

Independent Living Aids, Inc.
200 Robbins Ln.
Jericho, NY 11753
(800) 537-2118
(516) 937-1848
(516) 937-3906 Fax
http://www.independentliving.com
can-do@independentliving.com

IMPROVING MEMORY AND CONCENTRATION

230. **Write yourself reminder notes and put them where you'll see them.** For instance, if you have an appointment in the morning, tape a reminder note to the bathroom mirror so you will see it first thing.

231. **Set an alarm on your computer, microwave, watch, or pager to remind you to take medications, to drink or eat something, or to exercise.** Leave a note on the alarm or the computer so you know what to do when you turn off the alarm.

232. **To help with time and sequencing, create a calendar for the month with large squares for each day.** Then write down appointments, special events, and symbols for the weather in the appropriate square.

233. **To keep track of daily events, purchase a spiral notebook.** Start a new page for each day. Begin the day by recording the time of day and what happened. For example: "8:00 Breakfast (French Toast); 9:00 Talked to sister Ann."

234. **Keep your memory active by reviewing the day's news events with a friend or neighbor.** Read the daily newspaper together and then quiz each other on details of the stories that most interest you.

235. **To remember whether or not you have locked the door say out loud, "I'm locking the door" as you lock up.**

236. **We often think of things that we need to remember at inopportune times,** like in a darkened movie theater or out walking the dog. If it's inconvenient to write yourself a note, take off your watch or wedding band and put it on the opposite hand, or double-knot your shoelaces. That way, you will be reminded of the task and can make a note of it at a more convenient time. Give yourself a reminder that there is something you want to remember.

CHAPTER 7

Handling Medical Issues

Few of us are prepared for the diagnosis of a serious chronic illness like Parkinson's disease. However, as the reality of the diagnosis begins to take hold, you quickly learn that healthcare providers and medical professionals will now be a part of your life. Dealing with doctors, pharmacists, and therapists—not to mention all the new medical terminology, procedures, and tests—can be a real challenge. Keeping organized and taking an active role in managing your health care will give you back some control over your illness and assure family members that you are coping well with your new reality.

Managing your medical care will be easier if all your doctors and specialists belong to the same medical practice or HMO, because all your medical records will be in one place. In addition, seeing other specialists in the group (orthopedists, physiatrists, occupational/physical therapists, speech/language pathologists, and psychologists/psychiatrists) can reduce the hassles of obtaining referrals and filling out endless paperwork at new doctors' offices. Find out, too, if your insurance covers home health services for medical management in the home, physical therapy visits, and so on. You may be surprised at what is covered.

A healthcare provider's bedside manner can be extremely important. Choose a doctor whom you like and with whom you have a good rapport. Research shows that patients who are satisfied with their physicians are healthier overall than those who are not. If a friend or acquaintance recommends a doctor, keep in mind that you may have a different experience, opinion, or preference. If your doctor doesn't treat you with respect, listen to you, or see you as a whole person — as an individual, a family member, a person with a career and a social life— find one who does. Obtain a copy of the Patient's Bill of Rights and make sure your healthcare providers adhere to it. Learning to stick up for yourself and be your own advocate can give you back some of the power and control that PD takes away.

Another way to get involved in your own healthcare is to learn more than you ever wanted to know about PD. The American Parkinson's Disease Association (APDA) and the National Parkinson Foundation (NPF) are wonderful resources for accurate, up-to-date information. Enlist your friends and family members to do research, too, and collect information from newspapers, magazines, and medical journals. Visit a medical-school library if there is a university near your home, or search for reputable resources on the Internet. Share information and learn together. It will give you all something positive to do. You may find that you've read medical journal articles before your doctor has had a chance to read them. Bring the articles to your next appointment so you can discuss the findings and see how they relate to your case.

Be sure you and your family know how any prescribed medications work, what the side effects are, and which side effects you should report to your doctor. Do not take any medication, including nonprescription products, such as vitamins, dietary supplements, allergy and cold medicines, pain relievers, or herbal remedies, without first consulting your doctor.

This chapter contains many more tips and ideas to help you manage your medical care.

RECORD KEEPING AND RESEARCH

237. **Compile your own personal medical file.** Purchase a three-ring binder and several sheets with divider tabs. Use a three-hole punch so you can insert any kind of paper into the notebook. Organize the binder into sections:

◊ **Family health history.**

◊ **Past illnesses.**

◊ **Dated summaries of office appointments, tests, treatments, surgical procedures, and hospitalizations,** including copies of test results.

◊ **Prescription log,** with details about the names and dosages of all your medications, including nonprescription medications and vitamin supplements, and notes on why, when, and how often you take the drugs.

◊ **Symptom log,** to track how you feel before and after the introduction of a new medication, as well as recording any new symptoms or side effects. Keeping a symptom log is important because if you don't write them down, you may report only those symptoms to the doctor that you actually feel while you're in the office for an appointment.

◊ **Question and answer log,** to keep track of questions you have for your doctor, along with the answers you receive.

As the years pass, the file will be an invaluable reference. Keep it up to date and thorough. Bring it with you to all medical appointments, especially to your first appointment with a new doctor. The file doesn't take the place of your original medical records but it will help doctors get a quick overview and a thorough understanding of your history of treatment.

238. **Get copies of all your official medical records** and keep them in a special section of your personal medical file. More than half the states have enacted laws giving patients access to their hospital and physician records. You may have more difficulty elsewhere, but no state specifically denies access to your records. The cost to obtain your medical records may vary from state to state. Keep all medical documents in a central location where they can be easily found, and let family members and helpers know where the file is in case it is needed in an emergency.

239. **Carry an index card in your purse or wallet with a list of your medications** (including dosages), and any allergies or special medical conditions you have. You will be asked for this

information over and over again, and having it on paper is better than relying on memory. Use a second card for names and phone numbers of your primary care physician, your specialists, nurses, medical supply company, clergy, emergency contacts, etc. Carry both cards at all times. Also consider keeping this information in a small electronic planner or handheld personal data assistant (e.g., a Palm Pilot or Hewlett-Packard Jornada). Give a duplicate set of these cards to your helpers, family members, or close friends.

DOCTORS' APPOINTMENTS

240. **Mornings and right after the lunch hour are often the best times for scheduling a doctor's appointment.** At those times appointments are more likely to be running closer to schedule. Also consider the time of day you are most energetic, or when your medication leaves you at your peak.

241. **If you are anxious to see the doctor soon,** tell the receptionist and ask if there is an early opening due to a cancellation. If not, ask to be notified if someone does cancel. Then call back in a few days if you have not heard from the receptionist. Ask to be put on the "short list."

242. **If you have a lot to talk about with your doctor, make a consultation appointment** so the doctor will allow enough time to meet with you without being hurried. Give the receptionist the option of lengthening your appointment or scheduling a second appointment slot for you. You should be willing to pay for this extra time.

243. **Be clear about what you want to say to the doctor,** and try not to introduce extraneous information into your description of symptoms or other concerns. Write down your points in advance. It can be helpful to prepare a brief but accurate progress report, answering such questions as: How closely have you been following your treatment plan? How have you been feeling? How many hours a day do you feel "on" and "off?" Have you had any specific problems? What has been happening in your life? You may also want to have a family member or helper contribute to your progress report, recording their perceptions of your "on" and "off" times. Having more than one perspective can often give the physician a clearer picture. Remember, your doctor sees you only for a short amount of time. In order to adequately manage your PD, he or she needs to know how things have gone at home since your last appointment.

244. **Pay careful attention to your sleep patterns.** If you tend to fall asleep during a particular activity, tell your doctor. You might be experiencing sleep attacks, which are different from normal sleepiness. Also keep track of any hallucinations or delusions you might be experiencing. Medications can sometimes cause nocturnal wanderings, hallucinations, delusions, or other problems. Adjusting your dosage of a particular medication, or adding a new prescription, might help with those symptoms. If your sleep is still disturbed even after following your doctor's recommendations about the timing of your medication doses, consider getting an examination by a sleep spe-

cialist trained in managing patients with neurologic disorders.

245. **Bring pen and paper and write down what your doctor says.** Remembering everything your doctor advises can be a challenge. Sometimes it can be helpful to bring someone with you to the doctor's appointment to serve as a second set of ears. However, that strategy won't work if you feel unable to speak as freely to your doctor when a friend or family member is present. If you do bring someone along, be sure to communicate openly and honestly with your doctor.

246. **Ask for clarification** if for any reason you are not satisfied with the explanations your doctor gives you. If your doctor uses medical terms you do not understand, or if you are not sure how serious your diagnosis is, say so. Say, for example, "Could you say that in layman's terms?" or "I'm not sure I understood that. Would you explain it again?" If you wish to hear another opinion, ask for a second opinion from another physician. Don't worry about hurting your doctor's feelings; any reasonable practitioner should understand your desire to cover all the bases. Trust your instincts.

247. **If you have a medical test, protect yourself and your family by asking questions:** Are the tests processed in the office or are they sent out to an off-site lab? How long will it take to get the results back? When can you expect a call? Can you get a copy of the test results to keep in your home medical file? If you don't hear from the

doctor in the specified time, call until you get the information you need. Don't assume that "no news is good news." Sometimes test orders can be misplaced or delayed, so even if the doctor's office says they will contact you with the results, take the initiative yourself to find out the results.

248. **If your doctor recommends a particular treatment,** ask to be put in touch with other PD patients who have undergone the same treatment, or discuss it in a PD support group with others. Find out how effective it was and whether they had any adverse reactions to it.

MEDICATIONS

249. **Always ask your doctor or pharmacist for published information (a brochure from the manufacturer, for example) on any drug you've been prescribed.** If you have trouble reading printed material such as a prescription medication insert, enlarge it. Photocopy machines at copy shops, libraries and post offices are capable of enlarging print to make it easier to read. Or, use a magnifying glass to help you read.

250. **Ask specifically about every drug's side effects,** the amount of time it will take for the drug to reach full effectiveness in your body, and whether there are any potentially harmful interactions between the drugs you are taking (both prescription and nonprescription). Ask if you can try a one-week supply of the drug to see how well you tolerate it before purchasing an entire month's supply.

251. **Ask your doctor or pharmacist to write the number of times a day you should take your medication.** It is easy to misinterpret dosing instructions when they are written as hourly intervals (e.g., one tablet every six hours). But few people misinterpret instructions that specify daily frequency (e.g., one tablet four times per day). Write out the dosage schedule and carry it with you. Check off each dose as you take it. If a particular drug must be taken in the middle of the night, ask if there is an alternative prescription that is more convenient to take.

252. **Familiarize yourself with some of the abbreviations used on prescriptions:**

    ◊ QD=every day;

    ◊ BID=two times per day;

    ◊ TID=three times per day;

    ◊ QID=four times per day;

    ◊ PO=by mouth;

    ◊ AC=before meals;

    ◊ PC=after meals;

    ◊ HS=at bedtime.

253. **Choose one pharmacy to fill all of your prescriptions** to ensure that there will be an accurate record of all the medications you're taking. Also, find out if your pharmacy has a computer system that will automatically generate alerts when any of your prescriptions have harmful interactions.

254. **Ask your pharmacist for nonchildproof bottles with easy-open caps** if you have trouble opening traditional prescription bottles. Some pharmacies also offer large-print labels that are much easier to read.

255. **Save time and energy by having your prescriptions mailed from the pharmacy to your home.**

256. **Keep a list of your daily medications taped to the refrigerator, microwave, or medicine cabinet.** List the time of day, name of the drug, and dose. Check off each dose as you take it.

257. **Use a weekly pill organizer with morning and evening slots for each day.** At the beginning of each week, fill the organizer with your medications. You can also use a clean egg carton to organize your pills.

258. **Keep track of medication times by using one of the following methods:**

    ◊ **Purchase a digital sports watch with a countdown repeat timer** if you need to take medication every four hours, for example. With this feature, the watch beeps after four hours, then automatically starts counting down to the next four-hour interval. These watches come in men's and women's styles with metal or nylon bands. If you don't want to be disturbed by the watch beeping in the middle of the night, take it off and leave it in another room.

    ◊ **Purchase a "double alarm" alarm clock.** Because morning pills and evening pills are the easiest to remember, set the alarm to go off, for example, at 12:00 p.m. and 4:00 p.m. After the alarm rings at 4:00 p.m., press the reset button and the alarm will automatically sound the next day at 12:00 p.m.

259. **Take a hard-to-swallow pill with a spoonful of applesauce or pudding.** For more tips on making swallowing pills easier, see the section on swallowing in the *Managing Mealtime Madness* chapter.

260. **Be sure to discuss the specifics of pill splitting with your doctor.** Sometimes your doctor might prescribe a dosage that is smaller than what is commercially available and instruct you to split pills in half. Or, to save you money, your doctor might prescribe a higher dosage than you need and recommend that you split the pills. Another reason you might want to split pills is if certain pills are too large to swallow easily. Do not split or crush up hard-to-swallow pills without first checking with your physician. If you split pills, you can lose up to 20 percent of the pill's mass as dust and fragments (even if you use a pill-splitter). Be sure to ask your doctor if the effectiveness of the medicine would be diminished if 10 percent-20 percent of the medication were lost. If you still have to split pills, split them one at a time, as you need them. The rough edges of split pills will erode and lose even more of the medication if they are put back in the bottle.

261. **Never use household silverware to administer medication.** You could be receiving an incorrect dosage. Always use an oral dropper, cylindrical dosing spoon, syringe, or plastic

medicine cup. You can find these devices at a pharmacy or discount department store.

262. **Talk to your doctor if you are troubled by a dry mouth.** Many medications and medical conditions can cause dry mouth syndrome. Normal amounts of saliva are important to maintain healthy teeth and gums. Lack of it increases the incidence of decay and periodontal disease (gum disease). Also, saliva aids in swallowing, digestion, and the ability to speak normally. Because dry mouth is very common, products have been developed for the treatment of this condition. Many of these are sold over the counter in drugstores. Consult your doctor or dentist to discuss this common condition and possible treatments appropriate for you. In the meantime, keep a glass of water nearby and sip from it regularly during the day, swishing the water around in your mouth to moisten your gums.

263. **Tell your doctor if you experience dramatic changes in your mood** during the day, or from day to day. As many as fifty percent of people with PD have mood swings. Mood swings can be caused by the disease itself or by medications. Your doctor might alter your medications or recommend that you exercise regularly, start a new project, get involved in a support group, or talk with a therapist.

264. **Keep track of how you feel after eating various kinds of meals, and discuss with your doctor any dietary restrictions you should observe while on your medications.** The effectiveness of some PD medications is affected by diet. For

example, the absorption of levodopa is delayed if it is taken with a meal rich in protein. On the other hand, many people do not tolerate levodopa on an empty stomach and they experience nausea and vomiting. If taking medications causes nausea, try taking it with ginger ale or a gingersnap cookie.

265. **If you are taking Sinemet® try dissolving in a sugared, carbonated beverage** like Sprite™, Coca-Cola™, or ginger ale to optimize its effectiveness.

266. **If you are staying in the hospital, ask your doctor to write an order for you to be able to take your own Parkinson's disease medications.** This is important because sometimes it's difficult to get medication administered exactly on time while you are in the hospital. Generally, if medication is scheduled to be given at 1:00 P.M., it can be administered between 12:00 noon and 2:00 P.M. and still be considered on time. For people with PD, 10 to 15 minutes can be the difference between staying "on" and going "off." If you're admitted to a general medical unit, ask to speak with the head nurse about the importance of timing your PD medications to control your symptoms. Give the doctors and nurses a copy of your normal medication regime. Make sure a note is recorded in your chart so that you can give yourself your medications when you need them.

✍ Helping Hands

267. **If the person with PD begins hallucinating,** try to explain that the medicine isn't working

and is causing the hallucination. Keep notes on what time of day the hallucinations occur. Also record what was taken and when the medications were last taken. This will help the doctor if the medications need to be adjusted. Adjusting the medications may not make the hallucinations disappear, but they may be less disturbing. For example, if the person sees large green giants, medication adjustment may cause the person to see little green ants.

MANAGING YOUR HOME HEALTH CARE

268. **Buy a digital thermometer, not a glass one.** Digital thermometers are easier to read, and they are safer than glass because they won't break in your mouth.

269. **Use a microwaveable heat pad for backaches;** they are safer to use than electric heating pads. They cool down gradually like a hot water bottle and won't burn the skin.

270. **Wrap a Chux™ pad, a plastic-backed pad with an absorbent cotton lining typically used in bed for incontinence, around a warm compress.** The compress will stay warmer and the moisture won't seep out onto garments or furniture. You can purchase Chux™ or similar pads at drug stores.

271. **To make a cold compress,** wet a washcloth and keep it in a storage bag in your freezer. When you need a compress, remove it from

the freezer and allow it to thaw slightly. Then place it where you need it. When you have finished, just return the damp washcloth to the freezer.

272. **Use an inflatable neck cushion** to rest your head while lying in bed or sitting in your arm-chair. A U-shaped or dog bone-shaped pillow may also provide you with comfortable neck support.

👍 **Helping Hands**

273. **Use pillows to position the person with PD on his or her side in bed.** Therapists can show you how. Instead of buying big pillows, roll up towels and hold the roll in place with rubber bands. These towel pillows can be laundered easily, unlike large pillows.

👍 **Helping Hands**

274. **Create a makeshift backrest** for the person who must stay in bed and would like to sit up. First, remove the pillows from the bed. Then take a straight-backed chair and turn it upside down and place it where the pillows were. The front edge of the seat will touch the mattress and the legs of the chair will be up in the air near the headboard or wall. The top portion of the back of the chair will also touch the mattress creating a slanted surface on which you place the pillows to lean on.

275. **If you have leg cramps** a quick way to relieve them is to bite your lower lip while pinching

your upper lip. It may look silly, but it helps some people.

276. **If your arms feel cold,** pull a pair of children's leg warmers up your arm all the way to the underarm and shoulder. If your legs are cold, purchase a pair of adult-size leg warmers for your legs and knees. If your feet are cold in bed, wear regular short sport socks. If the elastic around the ankle is too tight, clip it to relieve any constriction.

277. **If you use a wheelchair or a scooter,** try out different wheelchair cushions until you find the one that is most comfortable for you. Consult your physical therapist for recommendations, and spend some time in your hospital's home health or rehab store trying out different cushions.

278. **To relieve constipation:**

◊ **Drink at least eight 8-ounce glasses of water every day.**

◊ **Add one cup of unprocessed bran cereal to your daily diet.** Or add bran powder to non-bran cereals, applesauce, or soup.

◊ **Sit comfortably on a low commode with knees drawn up** to help the abdominal muscles pass the stool.

◊ **Discuss other possible remedies with your doctor,** because the frequent use of laxatives, suppositories, and enemas can cause additional health problems.

RESOURCES

279. **If you are concerned about your safety** or the safety of someone else around the house, you may want to consider a service like Lifeline.® Lifeline® operates over a telephone line and is a 24-hour emergency response system service provided by most community hospitals. It utilizes a communicator unit that is hooked up to your phone, plus a portable help button you wear at all times. When you push the button, two-way communication between you and the Response Center is immediately activated through the powerful speakerphone in the communicator unit. When you subscribe to Lifeline® service, you provide a list of people to be contacted in case of an emergency. The staff at the Response Center has your list on file, and when you activate the help button, they ask the nature of the problem and whom you wish them to contact, or if you need emergency medical assistance. Check your local hospital to find out if a program like Lifeline® is available in your area.

280. **Paying for the high cost of drugs can be a serious problem for some people.** But now there are services that help people of any age, people with disabilities, and people with low incomes locate the Patient Assistance Programs offered by many pharmaceutical companies. These programs provide free medication to people who qualify. The Medicine Program is a volunteer organization that works in cooperation with the physician to assist patients who may qualify to enroll in one or more of the many Patient Assistance Programs available nationwide.

The Medicine Program
P.O. Box 515
Doniphan, MO 63935-0515
(573) 996-7300
http://www.themedicineprogram.com

281. **Use your computer to access the Internet to search for medical information.** The U.S. National Library of Medicine (NLM) allows you to search multiple databases for information on clinical trials, drugs, doctors, hospitals and healthcare facilities. Other databases list scientific journal articles and list consumer health libraries across the country.

U.S. National Library of Medicine
http://www.nlm.nih.gov

282. **To purchase home medical supplies,** check the Yellow Pages in your phone book for listings under First Aid Supplies, Medical Supplies, Surgical Appliances, and Physicians and Surgeons — Equipment & Supplies. Usually the kinds of outlets that offer home medical supplies are pharmacies, home health care stores (often affiliated with local hospitals), and surgical supply stores. You can also find many items in medical supply catalogs or online stores such as:

Unlimited Living, Inc.
P.O. Box 1499
Shepherdstown, WV 25443
(866) 222-4447
(304) 876-1490 Fax

http://www.unlimitedliving.com/
help@unlimitedliving.com

Allegro Medical
7342 E. Thomas Rd, Suite C.
Scottsdale, AZ 85251
(800) 861-3211
http://www.allegromedical.com/
feedback@AllegroMedical.com

RehabMart.com: Discount Rehab Superstore
150 Sagewood Drive
Winterville, GA 30683-1563
(800) 827-8283
(706) 213-1144
(603) 843-2144 Fax
http://www.rehabmart.com/

Smith & Nephew, Inc.
Rehabilitation Division
N104-W13400 Donges Bay Rd.
P.O. Box 1005
Germantown, WI 53022
(800) 558-8633
(262) 251-7840
(800) 545-7758 Fax
http://www.smith-nephew.com/us/rehab/
rehab.customercare@smith-nephew.com

283. **If you need special medical equipment for only a short time,** look into borrowing the equipment from local sources. Contact agencies like the Red Cross, Salvation Army, Visiting Nurse Service, home health agencies, churches, senior centers, and your local APDA chapter.

CHAPTER 8

Getting Out and About

Don't let Parkinson's disease (PD) limit your world. Take a few minutes to think over the errands you have to run before you leave the house. Is it a good time of day to be going to the library or post office? Will the drive-up windows at the bank be open? Rearrange the order of your stops to make errands most convenient for you. If you're prone to forget the sequence, write it down. Leave low-priority stops at the bottom of the list, so if you get tired you can leave them for another time.

Parkinson's disease and some of the medications used to control it can impact your perception and reaction time, and possibly affect your ability to drive safely. Be realistic about your abilities. Have someone else drive you if necessary. Discuss with a doctor your concerns about driving and see if adjusting your medications can improve your ability to drive.

With a little extra planning, a realistic itinerary, and some creativity, you can still get out and do many of the things you want to.

ERRANDS AND OUTINGS

284. **Plan ahead before going out.** Put your credit card in an easily accessible place, get out the money you will need for using public transportation, and begin to make out a check if you feel it takes too much time to do in the checkout lane. Then all you have to do is sign the check and ask the cashier to fill in the amount. When you get home, use the store receipt to fill in the amount of the check in the ledger.

285. **Before going out, call ahead to the restaurant, movie theater, etc., and ask if the establishment is accessible (including the restrooms).** Ask about parking facilities, about which is the most convenient entrance, and so on. When you reach your destination, keep seating arrangements in mind. If you use a wheelchair, ask for a table instead of a booth. If you are going to a theater but have trouble moving to accommodate others trying to reach seats further into your row, try to sit in a front row, or reserve the end seat and wait until the entire row has been seated before you sit down.

286. **Use a walkie-talkie set so you are never out of touch** when you go shopping with friends or relatives in large stores and malls. Otherwise, it can be easy to lose track of each other.

287. **If your destination lacks convenient seating— such as a museum, park, shopping mall, etc. — bring your own.** Many camping equipment stores sell portable folding stools that you can take along on walks for rest stops. Some

models come with a shoulder strap and others have their own tote bag.

288. **Take individually wrapped moist towelettes (the antibacterial kind) when you go out.** They are good for easy cleanup when washroom sinks are inaccessible. Use them when you go out in public and have contact with shopping cart handles, door handles, and public phones — notorious havens for contagious germs. Another option is to use an antibacterial hand sanitizer. These germ-killing gels are great when soap and water are not available.

289. **If you are unable to shake hands using your right hand because of tremors, arthritis, or another condition, offer your left hand.** If you are unable to offer either hand, simply say, "You'll have to excuse me, I am unable to shake your hand. I offer a smile instead."

CAR AND DRIVING

290. **Find out if you qualify for a disabled parking permit or a disabled license plate** if you have health problems or your ability to walk is impaired. With the permit you can park your vehicle in specially designated parking spaces. In some areas you may also park at metered stalls without payment, and for longer than the posted time limit. Contact your state's Department of Motor Vehicles about obtaining disabled parking privileges. You'll need a signed statement from your physician verifying your need for a temporary or permanent

permit, and in some cases you must periodically recertify your disability.

☝ Helping Hands

291. **Doctors may not restrict driving privileges, even though you may feel it is unsafe for the person with Parkinson's disease to drive,** and it may be difficult for you to take the car keys away or deny the person the right to drive. If the person with PD applies for a handicapped parking permit or for disabled plates, he or she will be required to take a driver's test, and the Department of Motor Vehicles may then revoke the person's driving privileges.

292. **Vehicles with leather or vinyl seats are easier to get into and out of than those with cloth fabric seats.** One way to make sliding in and out of the seat easier is to place a large sheet of plastic, such as a garbage bag or a vinyl drop cloth, on the seat before sitting down.

TRAVEL

Traveling by Car

293. **Take along your personal disabled windshield placard when you travel.** Disabled parking permits are honored in most states and often you can use your placard on a rental car or in a car in which you are a passenger. However, some states do not honor disabled placards issued from another state. If you are traveling by car, contact the police department

in your destination city to find out about the local ordinances. If you forget to bring your permit with you, your only option may be to visit the nearest Department of Motor Vehicles office and request a temporary permit. Don't be surprised if they want to see a doctor's letter certifying your disability or medical condition.

294. **Keep an extra outfit in the car** in case you spill something on your clothing and need to change.

295. **Use a U-shaped inflatable neck pillow to prevent getting a stiff neck from sleeping while sitting up during long car trips.**

Traveling by Air

296. **When making airline reservations, let the ticketing agent know if you have any special needs.** Will you need assistance boarding the plane? Do you require a special meal (low-fat, vegetarian, kosher, etc.)? Do you need an electric cart to get to a connecting flight? Do you need to fly with your oxygen tank? Do you require special seating? For example, you might want an aisle seat near the restroom if you need to make frequent trips. If you need more legroom or have difficulty maneuvering into seats, ask to be assigned to a bulkhead seat, which are at the front of the cabin. These seats are typically reserved for travelers for special needs. Also, keep in mind that while on board, flight stewards will ask you to stow your cane or walker. Let them know in advance if you will need assistance getting up and around in the cabin.

297. **Remember that with heightened airport security, you must present a photo ID** (usually a driver's license) when checking in so that airport personnel can match your picture ID with the name on the ticket. If you do not have a valid driver's license because of a disability, obtain a picture ID from your state's Department of Motor Vehicles. There is often a small service charge to obtain a picture ID .

298. **Save energy by making use of the conveniences many airports have for travelers.** When you enter the airport, let a porter carry your bags. Ask the porter to call for a wheelchair. Start out with a porter whom you can pay to take you every step of the way. Ask in advance if the porter can assist you with your bags to the ticket counter and then take you to the gate. Once you reach the gate, tell the gate agent if you will need any assistance boarding or during the flight. When you reach your destination, ask the gate agent to call for a porter, and ask the porter to take you from the gate to the baggage carousel, and finally to the taxi stand. It may cost a few dollars but it is worth it.

299. **If you must travel with medication that needs to be refrigerated,** bring along a thermal lunch bag that will hold a few doses of the medication. Insert a cool pack into the bag until you can give it to a flight attendant to refrigerate. It is also a good idea to have a letter from your physician stating that you are taking medication and need to travel with syringes and needles.

Packing

300. **Use Hefty One-Zip™ bags (or similar zipper-slide plastic bags) to pack similar items** of clothing together, (undergarments in one bag; t-shirts in another) and zip halfway. Then sit on the bag or squeeze it so all the air comes out, and zip it tight. You'll find that you can pack your clothing in a smaller, more manageable suitcase.

301. **Taking along these items when you travel can really save the day:**

     ◊ **a collapsible cup and drinking straws.**

     ◊ **cellophane tape.**

     ◊ **paper clips.**

     ◊ **Zip-Loc® plastic bags.**

     ◊ **a small, folding suitcase.**

     ◊ **a tape measure.**

     ◊ **an extra wristwatch and pair of eyeglasses.**

     ◊ **a calculator.**

     ◊ **a small spiral notebook and pencil.**

     ◊ **a small flashlight.**

     ◊ **packets of instant coffee, creamer, sweetener, bouillon cubes, and instant soup.**

     ◊ **an electric water heater that heats up a cup of coffee or water.**

302. **Pack your prescriptions and other medications in your carry-on bag.** If you pack them in your suitcase and the airline misplaces your

luggage, you may be stranded without your medicine for at least 24 hours. Also, carry with you an index card with important medical information including your diagnosis, medications, and family and doctors' contact information in case of an emergency.

Staying at a Motel or Hotel

303. **Before you go on vacation, contact the hotel where you will be staying and speak with the concierge.** He or she can make dinner reservations, arrange for play tickets, and provide information about other sights to see that otherwise might be unavailable to you. The concierge service is free, but tips are appreciated.

304. **If you travel with a wheelchair, bring along a length of string that spans the width of your wheelchair, or a tape measure.** Before checking in at a hotel or motel, ask the desk clerk to take the string or measuring tape and use it to measure the width of the door to your room, the bathroom, and the hotel elevator (if applicable). If there is enough clearance, you can check into the hotel with confidence.

305. **When you check into a hotel or motel,** make up a card to leave at the front desk that contains the following information: your name, your room number, the dates of your stay, and a brief description of special assistance you might need in case of emergency. Such an "ability-alert" card will stand out and let hotel and emergency staff know that you need help.

Index